# Education for Community Health

*Building a Community of Learning for the 21st Century*

*Francis Sarr*

# Education for Community Health

*Building a Community of Learning for the 21st Century*

**Also by the author**

*Community-Oriented Education for Health Professionals: A Cultural Analysis Approach to Curriculum Planning (2013)*

# Education for Community Health

*Building a Community of Learning for the 21st Century*

**Francis Sarr**

CENMEDRA

Published by CENMEDRA – the Centre for Media and Development Research in Africa



First published in The Gambia in 2017 by CENMEDRA
www.cenmedra.org

ISBN: 9789983952506

Printed in England

Front cover design by Sadibou Kamaso

Layout design: Sainabou Fofana

Cover photo: Faculty and students, School of Medicine and Allied Health Sciences, University of The Gambia
www.cenmedra.org
info@cenmedra.org

# List of Figures, Tables and Boxes

## Figures



## Tables

## Boxes

# Dedication

*For my lovely granddaughters – Sukunda Toupan, Harriet Toupan and Janet Toupan - who are already teaching me new things about the changing world.*

# About the author

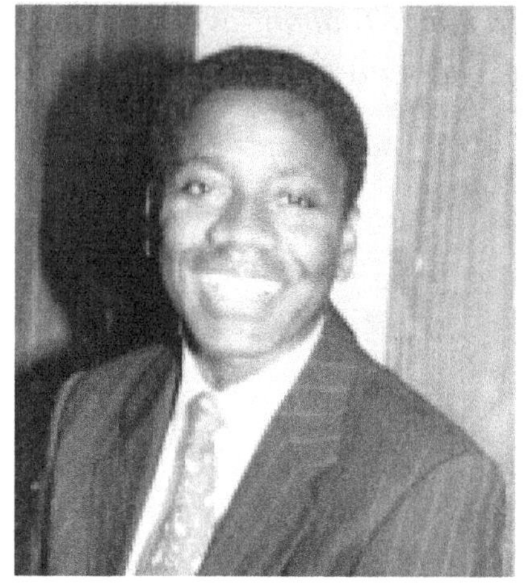

Francis Sarr, Associate Professor of Community Health Education and Fellow of the West African College of Nursing, is the Acting Dean of the School of Graduate Studies and Research of the University of The Gambia. He was educated at The Gambia School of Nursing and Midwifery (SRN Cert.); Pharmacy Department at The Gambia's Ministry of Health (Medical Aide Cert.); Cuttington University College, Liberia (BSc Nursing); University of Wales, Cardiff (M Ed, Curriculum Development & Educational Administration); London University School of Hygiene andTropical Medicine (MSc & Postgraduate Diploma, Public Health); London University Institute of Child Health (Nutrition & Child Health Cert.); and London South Bank University (PhD, Public Health).

He has a career in the health service that spans over a decade of working as a staff nurse and dispenser in urban and rural health services and 33 years of teaching in nursing and midwifery education. He participated in the planning of Primary Health Care (PHC) in The Gambia at headquarters and lower levels and was instrumental in the orientation of nursing and midwifery programmes to the PHC approach. A dedicated public health scholar and practitioner, Sarr is passionate about innovative approaches to healthcare education in the global South.

# Acknowledgements

I am grateful to the authors, theorists and experts from whom I have drawn inspiration – too many to mention here. I am especially thankful to my peer reviewers namely Dr Josiah Alamu of the University of Illinois, Springfield, USA; Professor Laura Serrant of the University of Wolverhampton, UK; Oyedunni Arologun, Associate Professor at the University of Ibadan, Nigeria; Dr Maria Horne of Bradford University, UK; and Matt Rietschel, associate professor at the University of Maryland, USA. I am also grateful to my students, both past and present; my editor Aloa Ahmed Alota; and all my colleagues in health care and at the University of The Gambia, who have in different ways helped deepen my knowledge and understanding of health care in general. Over and above all else, I am deeply appreciative of the support and care of my entire family, in particular that of my adoring wife – Antoinette.

# About CENMEDRA

CENMEDRA – the Centre for Media and Development Research in Africa – is a knowledge centre. Registered as an educational charity in The Gambia on 3 March 2014 it aims to promote, facilitate and disseminate research in media, communication and development in Africa. Its activities are focused on five main areas namely media research, researching development, new media and society, education, and publication. In line with its underlying aim of research application, it shares its research results with policymakers, media and development practitioners, media houses, regulators, scholars, politicians, librarians, activists, donors, development agencies, and the wider research community. It has a two-tiered governance structure: a board of trustees drawn from the media, civil society and academia, which provides strategy and policy direction, and an administrative secretariat that is responsible for operations and policy implementation.

## Mission

CENMEDRA exists to foster innovative research that puts Africa on the path of peace, progress and prosperity.

## Vision

CENMEDRA envisions an enlightened African society, free from the burden of ignorance, where everyone is able to realise their fullest potential in peace and prosperity.

## Values

- Integrity
- Openness
- Creativity
- Diligence

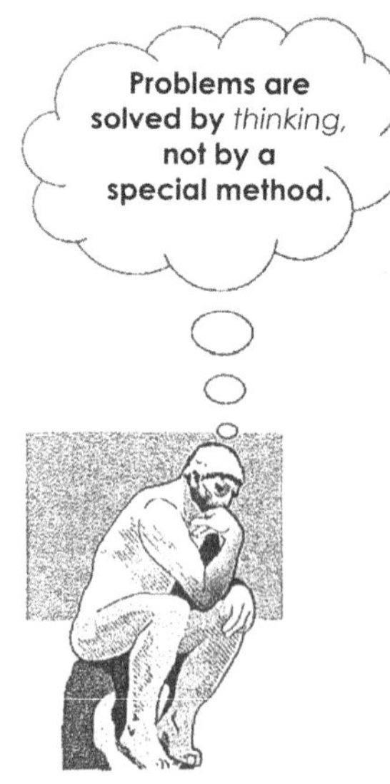


(Adapted from Thomas, G., 2011, p.6)

# Preface

This book aims primarily to demonstrate how faculty, students and communities can engage and learn from each other in order to build a community of learning and enhance teaching and learning through three strategic community processes (Bickford et al 2010): (i) designing learning spaces (ii) using information and communication technologies (ICTs), and (iii) designing pedagogy, curricula and co-curricular activities for learning. It describes how these three strategic community processes interact to build a community that fosters teaching and learning in community health. In doing so, it applies good practices to the design process and development of interventions that reflect the Primary Health Care (PHC) principles of self-reliance, equity, community participation and inter-sectoral collaboration (World Health Organisation – WHO - 1978). These principles are integrated into the practice of community health care at all levels: homes, dispensaries, health centres and hospitals. The premise interwoven through all three strategic community processes is developmental, which makes each process appropriate for community health education and practice. Thus, this book is about both community health and primary health care in relation to the idea of building a community of learning for community health.

Another aim of this book is to highlight the important role ICTs – supported cooperative and collaborative teaching and learning strategies can play in fostering a community of learning for community health and how community health educators can use these learning approaches to enhance such learning. While there may be other useful teaching and learning strategies for achieving this purpose, for example, students participating in class discussion, the cooperative and collaborative modes of teaching and learning are arguably the most important teaching and learning strategies for succeeding with this intent of building a community of learning for community health.

Using these approaches to learning in the community, students can form the social interactions needed to establish and build a community of learning for community health. They can create the notion of a community of learning in the absence of faculty involvement. Similarly, by using these learning frameworks, faculty can have a positive impact in shaping and extending the learning environment of students in the community. The ICTs-supported collaborative learning concept in particular enables students to build knowledge together (Dooly 2008), which deepens their education in community health and enables them to become more equipped to deal with the challenges they will meet after their education. Furthermore, ICTs-supported cooperative and collaborative teaching and learning reflects the push to prepare students to be responsible citizens in an increasingly technologically advanced world (Dooly 2008).

The book is divided into two interrelated parts, namely Part One and Part Two. Part One contains a set of theories, models, concepts and frameworks for a better understanding of the idea of building a community of learning in community health. Several of these theories, models and frameworks have been selected as examples of those that are found to be most useful. Some of them like the traditional educational theories are well known. Others like the community of learning concept and framework are relatively new in the literature. What one finds is that the theories, models, concepts and frameworks are interrelated. One cannot talk, for example, about building a community of learning in community health and primary health care without discussing motivation and leadership. Various theories, models, concepts and frameworks can be used to describe the same issues and developments. The aim of Part One therefore is to provide a language and linking concepts that are necessary for interpreting experience, to learn from others' experiences, as well as our own (Handy 1993). Part Two, on the other hand, demonstrates how such language can be used to assist with better comprehension of the issues that influence the building of a community of learning that need to be dealt with in the building process. It is an attempt to provide a comprehensive demonstration of how the language and concepts of Part One can be translated into actual actions directed at building a community of learning in community health.

# PART ONE

## *Concepts, Principles, Elements of Community Health and Primary Health Care*

# 1

## Community Health and Population Health
## A Comparative Analysis

Community means a group of people who live in a defined geographical location and are governed by the same rules and regulations, norms, values, goals and organisation. Its members are committed to interacting with one another broadly and honestly (Scott Peck et al 1993). It can set standards for members and create the environment for great achievements (Manning et al 1996).

The term community health means the health status of a defined group of people or community and the actions and conditions that protect and improve the health of the community (Green et al 2002). For instance, the health status of people living in a particular village and the actions taken to protect and improve their health constitutes community health. However, in addition to communities there are other groups that frequently need health care and are of relevance to policymakers. Therefore, the term population health has been proposed (Green et al 2002). However, according to Kindig et al (2003, p.1), this term is relatively new and has not been properly defined. They therefore propose this definition of population health: "The health outcomes of a group of individuals, including the distribution of such outcomes within the group." Kindig et al argue that the field of population health should include patterns of health determinants and health outcomes as well as policies and interventions that connect health determinants and health outcomes. Determinants of health include medical care systems (e.g., resource allocation and health interventions), the social environment (e.g., income, education and social support) and the physical surroundings (e.g., clean air and water, and urban design). Examples of health outcomes are longevity and health-related quality of life.

The term population health is similar to community health. The difference between population health and community health lies only in the scope of the people dealt with or the degree of organisation (McKenzie et al 2011). The health status of populations who are not organized or have no identity as a group or locality and the actions and conditions needed to protect and improve the health of these populations constitute population health (McKenzie et al 2011). Examples of populations are women over fifty years, adolescents, and adults between twenty-five and forty-four years of age, seniors living in public housing, prisoners, and blue-collar workers. It is clear from these examples that a population could be a segment of a community, a category of people in several communities of a region, or workers in various industries. The reader is referred to the wealth of literature around community and population for further exploration of the terms and concepts. Examples are Ruderman, M (2000) and Green et al (1999).

As health is influenced by a wide array of socio-demographic factors, relevant variables range from the proportion of residents of a given age group to the overall life expectancy of the neighbourhood. Medical interventions designed to improve the health of a community range from improving access to medical care to public health communications campaigns (Green et al 2012).

Currently, community health studies are focusing on how the built environment and socio-economic status affect community/population health. This is because there is growing evidence to show, for example, that physical and mental problems are linked to the built environment, including human places like homes, schools, workplaces and industrial areas (Srinivasan et al 2003). Such a research concentration is particularly relevant to building a community of learning in community health because it deals with the surroundings created by human beings for learning, such as buildings and neighbourhoods and their supporting infrastructure (e.g., water supply or energy networks). The built environment is a material, spatial and cultural product of human labour that combines physical elements and energy in forms suitable for living, working and playing. Practically, the built environment refers to the interdisciplinary field which addresses the design, construction, management and use of these man-made surroundings as an interrelated whole as well as their relationship to human activities over time. The following paragraphs show how and why this relates to community/population health.

The discipline draws upon areas such as economics, law, public policy, management, geography, design, technology, and environmental sustainability (Chynoweth 2006). The building of a community learning framework, as outlined in Chapter 7, is conceived as a development intervention and includes (1) learning space design (2) technology, community, and information exchange and (3) pedagogical, curricular, and co-curricular design. Thus, the implementation of the building of a community of learning framework can contribute significantly to community health education development.

As the WHO also suggests: The social conditions in which people live powerfully influence their chances to be healthy. Indeed factors such as poverty, social exclusion and discrimination, poor housing, unhealthy early childhood conditions and low occupational status are important determinants of most diseases, deaths and health inequalities between and within countries (WHO 2004, as cited by Dahlgren et al 1991).

Let us use the Dahlgren and Whitehead (1991) Social Model of Health (Figure 1) to help explain the layers of influence on community/population health and discuss inequalities in health based on socioeconomic position. In discussing the layers of influence on health, Dahlgren and Whitehead (1991) outline a social ecological theory to health. They try to map the relationship between individuals, their environment and disease.

**Figure 1: Dahlgren and Whitehead Social Model of Health (1991)**

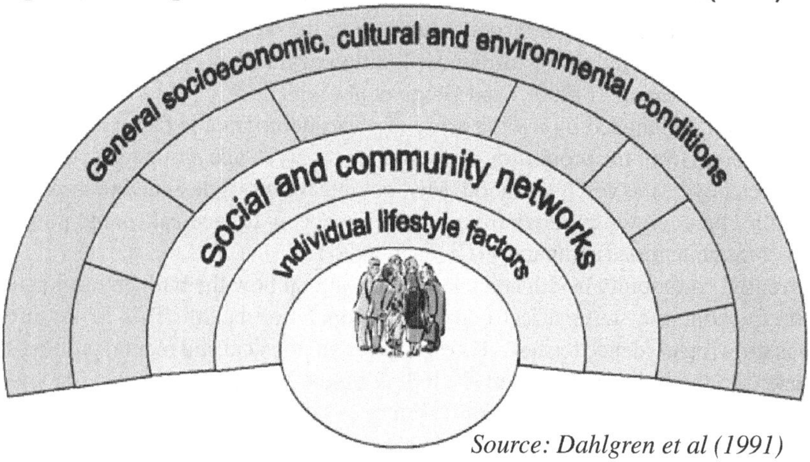

General socioeconomic, cultural and environmental conditions

Social and community networks

Individual lifestyle factors

*Source: Dahlgren et al (1991)*

**The model shows the following influences on community/population health:**

1. At the centre are individuals with a set of fixed genes. They are surrounded by influences on health that can be changed.
2. First layer is personal behaviour and lifestyle. These can promote or damage health, for example, choosing to drink alcohol or not. Here, individuals are affected by friendship patterns and the norms of their community.
3. Second layer is social and community influences, which provide mutual support for members of the community in unfavourable conditions. But they can also fail to provide support or have a negative effect.
4. Third layer includes structural factors, namely housing, working conditions, access to services and provision of essential facilities.

The model provides a useful framework for inquiring about the largeness of the contributions of each of the layers to health; the possibility of converting particular factors and the reciprocal actions needed to induce connected factors in other layers. Also, the model can be used for constructing several hypotheses on the inter-working between the different determinants of health, and the comparative influences of those determinants on various determinants (Public Health Action Support Group 2011).

In the introduction of their work entitled *European Strategies for Tackling Social Inequities in Health*, Dahlgren and Whitehead (2006) point to this relationship between the individual, his or her environment and disease, and the unfairness of health inequities, which they say are caused by unhealthy public policies and lifestyles influenced by structural factors. They highlight the importance given to efforts at reducing health inequities by an increasing number of countries and international bodies, such as some European Union countries and the WHO, and the importance of improving health generally, especially in low-income countries, through attempts by countries and international agencies like the Commission on Social Determinants of Health (WHO 2008). Dahlgren and Whitehead (2006) also point out that despite such efforts, there still remain many gaps that need to be filled. As they indicate, very few countries have developed particular strategies for integrating equity-oriented health policies into economic and social policies. Also, they say that the equity view is missing in many particular programmes that concentrate on various determinants of health, "even in those countries that claim that reducing social inequities in health is an overriding objective for all health-related policies and programmes". They further suggest that when one considers that people see health as composing one of the most significant dimensions of their welfare, the low priority it is accorded is disproportionate to its significance.

It is worth focusing further on the Commission on Social Determinants of Health (WHO 2008) as its recommendations, particularly those on education and training, have much relevance for building a community of learning for community health. The Commission on Social Determinants of Health was set up by the WHO in 2005 to arrange the evidence on what can be done to promote health equity, and to foster a global movement to achieve it. The Commission identified three principles of action which are included in three overarching recommendations, which the WHO sees as critical for achieving a more equitable and highest attainable standard of health. The three main principles are:

- Improve daily living conditions
- Tackle the inequitable distribution of power and money
- Measure and understand the problem and assess the impact of action

**Box 1: Recommendations for Training and Education of Medical and Health Professionals on the Social Determinants of Health**

- Educational institutions and relevant ministries make the social determinants of health a standard and compulsory part of training of medical and health professionals.
- The healthcare sector has an important stewardship role in inter-sectoral action for health equity.
- The recommended reorientation of the healthcare sector towards a greater importance of prevention and health promotion.
- Making the social determinants of health a standard and compulsory part of medical training and training of other health professionals requires that textbooks and teaching materials are developed for this purpose.

*Source: WHO (2008)*

The WHO (2008) offers several specific curriculum proposals on training and education of medical and health professionals on the social determinants of health together with the above recommendations:

- Medical and health professionals should be aware of health inequities as an important public health problem, and understand the importance of social factors in influencing the level and distribution of population health.
- Policymakers and professionals in the healthcare sector should understand how social determinants influence health, and how the healthcare sector, depending on its structure, operations, and financing, can exacerbate or ameliorate health inequities.
- Medical and health professionals need to be aware of how gender influences health outcomes and health-seeking behaviour.
- There should be reorientation in the skills, knowledge, and experience of the health personnel involved in disease prevention and health promotion and an enhancement of the professional status and importance of these areas.
- Textbooks and teaching materials should be developed for the purpose of making the social determinants of health a standard and compulsory part of medical training and training of other health professionals. This includes an urgent need to develop, among other things, a virtual repository of teaching and training materials on a broad range of social determinants of health that can be downloaded without cost.
- Opportunities for interdisciplinary professional training and research on social determinants of health should be created. For low-income countries, the creation of such training and education opportunities can happen, for example, through regional centres of learning and/or distance education models.

Like the WHO Report of the Commission on the Social Determinants of Health (WHO 2008), the Marmort Report (UCL Institute of Health Equity 2010), entitled Fair Society, Healthy Lives, focuses on proposing the most effective evidence-based strategies for reducing health inequalities, in this case in England from 2010. In doing so the report does a number of things:

- It proposes an evidence- based strategy to address the social determinants of health, the conditions in which people are born, grow, live, work and age and which can lead to health inequalities.
- It draws further attention to the evidence that most people in England are not living as long as the best off in society and spend longer in ill health. Preventable illnesses and premature death affect everyone below the top.
- It proposes a new way to reduce health inequalities in England post-2010.
- It argues that, traditionally, government policies have focused resources only on some segments of society. To improve health for all and to reduce unfair and unjust inequalities in health, action is needed across the social gradient.

Box 2 presents the key messages of the Marmot Report:

**Box 2: Key Messages of The Marmot Report**

1. Reducing health inequalities is a matter of fairness and social justice. In England, the many people who are currently dying prematurely each year as a result of health inequalities would otherwise have enjoyed, in total, between 1.3 and 2.5 million extra year of life.
2. There is a social gradient in health – the lower a person's social position, the worse his or her health.
3. Health inequalities result from social inequalities. Action on health inequalities requires action across all the social determinants of health.
4. Focusing solely on the most disadvantaged will not reduce health inequalities sufficiently.
   To reduce the steepness of the social gradient in health, actions must be universal, but with a scale and intensity that is proportionate to the level of disadvantage.
5. Action taken to reduce health inequalities will benefit society in many ways. It will have economic benefits in reducing losses from illness associated with health inequalities. These currently account for productivity losses, reduced tax revenue, higher welfare payments and increased treatment costs.
6. Economic growth is not the most important measure of our country's success. The fair distribution of health, well-being and sustainability are important social goals. Tackling social inequalities in health and tackling climate change must go together.
7. Reducing health inequalities will require action on six policy objectives:

- Give every child the best possible start in life.
- Enable all children, young people and adults to maximise their capabilities and have control over their lives.
- Create fair employment and good work for all.
- Ensure healthy standard of living for all.
- Create and develop healthy and sustainable places and communities.
- Strengthen the role and impact of ill-health prevention.

8. Delivering these policy objectives will require action by central and local government, the National Health Service (NHS), the private sectors and community groups. National policies will not work without effective local delivery systems focused on health equity in all policies.
9. Effective local delivery requires effective participatory decision-making at local level. This can only happen by empowering individuals and local communities.

*Source: UCL Institute of Health Equity 2014.*

As will be seen, many of these proposals, particularly those of the WHO Report of the Commission on the Social Determinants concerning training and education, are consistent with the major parts of this book, especially Chapters 5 and 9 on technology, community, information exchange and learning; Chapter 10 on pedagogy, curricular and co-curricular design; Chapter 11 on designing online co-operative and collaborative learning projects in community health; Chapter 12 on professional development in community health; and Chapter 13 on development of teaching and learning centres in community health. The frameworks that these chapters offer can assist community health educators who want to reorient the skills, knowledge, and experiences of community health personnel on the social determinants of health and enhance learning in community.

We must now consider the concept of PHC which is closely related to the idea of community/population health and the meaning of building a community of learning for community health.

**Principles and Elements of Primary Health Care**

Community health mainly in the contexts of developing countries is usually studied and delivered based on the PHC approach (e.g. Golladan (1980). Community health services play an important role in the primary health care system and aim to improve the health and well-being of people, especially people who are at risk of poorer health. Community health services provide a strong stage for the delivery of a range of primary health care services, such as child health services. If delivered effectively, a PHC system can improve the health of a population and reduce inequalities in health care (Department of Health 2014), which has been the focus of much of the foregoing discussion.

Members of the 13th World Health Assembly committed themselves to the PHC approach by adopting the resolution of "Health for All by the Year 2000" and define PHC thus:

> ...essential health care based on practical, scientifically sound and socially accepted methods and technology made universally accessible to individuals and families in the community through their full participation and at a cost that the community and country can afford to maintain at every stage of their development in the spirit of self-reliance and self-determination (WHO1978: 6).

The principles of PHC have been simplified thus: the health care services should be accessible to all; there should be maximum individual and community involvement in the planning and operation of health care services; the focus of care should be on prevention and promotion rather than on cure; appropriate technology should be used – that is, methods, procedures, techniques and equipment should be scientifically valid, adapted to local needs and acceptable to users and to those for whom they are used; health care is regarded as only a part of total health development - other sectors such as education, housing, nutrition are all essential for the attainment of a person's well-being.

Within the limits of this outline are eight important elements of a PHC service:

- Education on common health problems and ways to control and prevent them.
- Appropriate nutrition and improvement of food provision.
- Safe water supply and basic sanitation.
- Health care for mothers and children, incorporating family planning.
- Immunisation towards the main infectious diseases.
- Prevention and control of locally endemic diseases.
- Proper treatment of prevalent injuries and diseases.
- Supply of essential drugs (WHO 1978)

A PHC approach places emphasis on community-based services with increased attention to early intervention and prevention strategies such as health promotion. To be successful, community health programmes must depend on the dissemination of information by health professionals to the general public, using mass communication (one-to-one or one-to-many communication). Moreover, there is now a growing move towards health marketing (processes for creating, communicating, delivering, and exchanging offerings that have value for customers, clients, partners, and society at large) that combines traditional marketing principles and theories together with science-based strategies to prevention, health promotion and health protection (CDC 2011). Let us now look at the factors that contributed to the development of PHC in the past three decades.

**The Realities**

The effects of the dramatic social, political and economic changes such as liberal democratic systems, which came after the end of the Cold War and remained during the last ten years of the twentieth century, will continue to influence the daily lives of people globally in the 21st century in several ways. There will be continuous demands for social justice and respect for human rights, good governance, democracy, and a clear definition of the role of the state (WHO 1995). There will be enduring calls for the expansion of the involvement of communities in economic globalisation and decision-making (WHO 1995). Also, frequently there will be a need to adapt and change planned economies to market economies. Although the advantages of these changes are still unquestionable, clearly many countries are unable to make them in the medium-term due to socio-economic constraints and other factors.

The burden on governments to meet competing political, social and economic demands often results in the adoption of short-term reforms, which are usually far less effective (WHO 1995). In consequence, the drive towards immediate increased economic efficiency often leads to a reduction of funds for social programmes, in particular health care programmes (WHO1995). Although in many countries per capital income has increased in the last 40 years, many people are yet to experience improvements in quality of life, and many have suffered as a result of the changed processes (Shah 2013). For example, because of the structural adjustment policies of the World Bank and the International Monetary Fund (IMF), national governments are finding it increasingly difficult to ensure that their people get health care, food and education, which are basic human rights. Many developing countries have experienced deepening poverty and crippling debts as a result of such policies. Scores of people have been displaced, or are refugees; burdened or disadvantaged by unrestrained exploitation and war. War in turn has caused resource diversion and ruin in many parts of the world.

Several factors aggravate this situation in which governments are striving to meet competing social, economic and political demands. There is an increase in the total world population with the resultant pressure on health services. Additionally, not only has the number of poor people doubled in the last 15-20 years; but the gap between literate and illiterate people, rich and poor, in developed and developing nations is expanding (WHO 1995). This is seen more so in developing than in developed countries. During the 1960s, the income of 20 percent of the richest segment of the world's population was 30 times more than a similar number of the poorest segment (WHO 1995). This difference in income doubled in the 1990s. Moreover, the average consumption rate of natural resources in developed countries is 10-12 times that consumed by developing nations (WHO 1995). This widening gap between the rich and the poor, who cannot gain technology for development, represents the fundamental differences in today's world (Jeguier 1981).

The massive capital movement from industrialised countries to poor ones goes to countries with the capacity to provide large markets and export industrial material (WHO 1995). This is mainly due to private investment. Despite the important role technical cooperation and external aid play, the volume of bilateral assistance to the health sectors of poor countries has been dwindling. Government measures and economic adjustment programmes have proved to be ineffective alternatives for health development. Therefore, it is imperative that donors earmark adequate resources and other necessary requirements for sustainable development, poverty alleviation, relief and conflict resolution (WHO 1995).

It is clear from what is portrayed above that economic, political, environmental, social, and cultural factors were instrumental in the development of PHC in the past three decades. As information from the 1994 monitoring of the Health-for-All Strategy (cited in WHO1995) also indicates, these influences will remain the major determinants of health in the 21st century. These factors not only constitute the background for change that was formally expressed in 1978 at Alma-Ata; they also form the basis for the renewal of the Health-for-All Strategy (WHO 2014). Box 3 provides reasons given by the WHO for the renewal of the Health – for - All Strategy that reflects very much the social, economic, environmental and political realities described above.

**Box 3: Reasons for Renewal of the Health – for - All Strategy**

Why a renewal of primary health care (PHC), and why now, more than ever? The immediate answer is the palpable demand for it from Member States – not just from health professionals, but from the political arena as well.

Globalisation is putting the social cohesion of many countries under stress, and health systems, as key constituents of the architecture of contemporary societies, are clearly not performing as well as they could and as they should.

People are increasingly impatient with the inability of health services to deliver levels of national coverage that meet stated demands and changing needs, and with their failure to provide services in ways that correspond to their expectations. Few would disagree that health systems need to respond better – and faster – to the challenges of a changing world. PHC can do that.

*Source: WHO (2014)*

However, what are the implications of pursuing this direction for health professional education in the 21st century? We will consider this question in Chapter 2 by looking at the proposed changes in curricula required for primary health care and community health. In the next section, we will consider important PHC reforms since the initiation of the PHC approach.

**PHC Reforms**

Primary health care reforms have been discussed and proposed in many different countries since members of the 13th World Health Assembly adopted the resolution of "Health for All by the Year 2000". The expectations of Health-for-All had led countries to formulate different models of health care towards such a goal during recent decades, creating opportunities that have stimulated a series of new health concepts and paradigms. In The Gambia, for example, PHC was adopted in 1979 as the basis for the provision of essential health care and became an integral component of development programmes.

The PHC approach in The Gambia aimed at mobilising all potential resources, including the communities' own resources, towards the development of a national health care system. The intention was to extend health service coverage to the entire Gambian population and to tackle the main disease problems of the communities. PHC is also a mechanism for guaranteeing an equitable re-distribution of the limited health resources available in the country in favour of the underserved majority who live and work in rural areas (MOH 1981).

There are many conceptions on which the principles and concepts of PHC are based (e.g, Bhatia et al 2010). One such example is the conceptualisation of Community-based Integrated Care (Plochg et al 2002), which features a health system that is based upon and driven by community health needs. Moreover, it is tailored to the health beliefs, preferences, and societal values of that community and assures a certain level of community participation. Recently, this approach was renewed by introducing terms such as responsiveness and stewardship. Another example is Community-Oriented Primary Care, defined as a "continuous process by which primary health care is provided to a defined community on the basis of its assessed health needs through the planned integration of public health practice with the delivery of primary health care" (Mullan et al 2002, p 1748). Mullan et al provide a global overview of COPC, tracing its conceptual roots, reviewing its many manifestations, and exploring its prospects as an organisational paradigm for the democratic organisation of community health services. They examine the pitfalls and paradoxes of the concept and suggest its future utility.

A main belief of the renewed push for PHC, as suggested by Gofin et al (2005), is that community medicine and primary health care are actually a component of a unified practice, pointing out the relationships between PHC and community-oriented primary care (COPC): a comprehensive approach that identifies health needs or problems; taking into account socio-economic and cultural factors that determine health, and providing health care to a whole community. While these conceptions of health care may vary somewhat in their meanings, what they all clearly have in common is the emphasis that the concepts of PHC should be integrated into the practice of community health care in homes, dispensaries, health centres and hospitals, which constitute the different levels of health care.

Most definitions of PHC in relation to a renewed primary health care system would have the following characteristics:

- More community-based PHC organisations focus on the specific needs of the individuals and populations that they serve.

- Greater coordination and integration with other health services, for example, hospitals and home care services.

- A greater emphasis on health promotion, illness and injury prevention and the management of chronic diseases, to help people stay healthy and not just focus on treatment once they are sick.

- Care provided by a team of primary health care providers (for example, nurses, family,physicians, nutritionists, counsellors, just to name a few) so that the most appropriate care is provided by the most appropriate provider.

- Greater access to health services, on a 24/7 basis, so that people can get advice and care outside of regular office hours.

In order to meet the requirements of 'a renewed primary health care system' professionals will be required to collaborate to develop comprehensive care plans (e.g. WHO 2014). This will require professionals to take the time to get to know the skills that different professional groups bring to the PHC setting. Not only will PHC teams be challenged to incorporate various approaches through which to see clients, they will also be challenged to develop an understanding of, and responsiveness to, the changing needs of the communities they serve.

On a more macro level, a genuine PHC approach will require governments to take into account the physical, social and economic factors that impact upon individuals and shift the focus away from treating illness to broader social health focus to tackle inequalities in health. The World Health Organisation has identified five areas for action (Box 4):

**Box 4: A Renewed PHC System: Five Areas for Action**

- build healthy public social policy
- create supportive environments
- strengthen community action
- re-orient health services
- develop individual personal skills

*Source: WHO (1987)*

One of the challenges posed by Bhatia et al (2010), for example, concerning the renewed push for PHC is moving away from a narrow technical bio-medical paradigm of health to a broader social determinants approach and the need to differentiate primary care from primary health care. The difference between the meaning and the appropriate use of the concepts of "primary health care" and "primary care" has been further explained by, for instance, the Report of the Canadian National Primary Health Care Conference (Lewis et al 2004). According to the report, primary care deals mainly with the prevention and treatment of sickness. It is what many people think of as front-line care. Conventionally, this takes the form of a visit to the family doctor. Primary care may involve preventative activities, immunisation, diagnosis and treatment of illness. However, such care does not usually include a comprehensive, intersectional approach to producing or enhancing health. Perhaps most crucially, primary care concentrates on individuals and families, but not the community as the unit of intervention which, as we have seen in the explanation above, is one of the hallmarks of the primary health care approach. Nevertheless, primary care is an essential subset of primary health care. They are complementary, and neither can be effective or efficient without the other. Thus, the idea of education for community health, as used in this book, incorporates both conceptions of primary care and primary health care.

**Summary**

This chapter has looked at the concepts, principles and elements of community health and the primary health care approach on which the implementation of community health in the developing country context is usually based. Community health is a discipline that deals with the health status of a defined and organised group of people, or community, and the actions and conditions that protect and improve the health of the community. A similar concept, population health, means the health status of populations who are not organised or have no identity as a group or locality and the actions and conditions needed to protect and improve the health of these populations. Many healthcare concepts rest on the principles and ideas of PHC and Community Health. For example, there is the idea of Community-based Integrated Care, which features a health system that is based upon and driven by community health needs.

However, much more than policy statements and dedicated resources are required to advance the needed shift in thinking away from institutional models and the emphasis on the treatment of illness. To meet the needs of 'a renewed primary health care system' professionals will, for instance, be required to collaborate to develop comprehensive care plans. There are several challenges on the renewed push for PHC, such as moving away from a narrow technical bio-medical paradigm of health to a broader social determinants approach and the need to differentiate primary care from primary health care. These two concepts are, however, reciprocal and are required for an efficient PHC/Community Health system. The following chapters deal with ideas about education and learning, management and building a community of learning for educating health professional in community health and PHC.

# 2

# *Educational Theories, Ideologies and Focus on the Community*

This chapter must necessarily start by making the point that there is no universal agreement on the meaning of the term education. The debate on what education actually means is as relevant to building a community of learning in community health education as it is in other areas of education. Many of the factors that diminish community of learning, such as the stress on the production-oriented approach to education that is characterised by larger class sizes, may be based on the varying understandings of what education signifies. This chapter therefore will first critically look at the principal theories and ideologies of education in the literature to structure a practical philosophy that will fit the process of building a community of learning for community health. It will then consider the educational focus on the community that is influenced by the fundamental principles and elements of community health and PHC.

## Dominant Theories of Education

There have been three dominant but contrasting views in education, examples of which are identifiable by the different ways education is loyally and devotedly delivered in educational institutions for health professions. The main features and assumptions of each are outlined as follows:

### Traditional Education (Subject-matter centred)

**Main features**

- Looks to the past for its content and ideas.
- Maintains its identity through an effort to conserve and transmit the heritage of the past.
- Organises and presents subject-matter in a logical method.
- Prepares one ineffectively for the solution of problems and continuous adjustment to change.

**Main assumptions**

- Cooperation.
- Respect for law, honesty, trustworthiness, and thrift.
- Regard for the other person's rights and feelings.
- Loyalty to family, church, government.

**Progressive Education (Child-centred)**
**Main features**

- The teacher is a guide whose duty is to observe the spontaneous activities of the learner and to study their mental and emotional reactions.
- Content and activities are selected to further the immediate purposes of children.
- Experience in meeting new situations prepares learners for future needs.
- A try-out for meeting situations later in life.
- Not all teachers are artist teachers and not all schools' situations are ideal.

**Main assumptions**

- Content and activity should be selected because of their inherent importance to students; this includes traditional subject-matter that connects definitely with the problem at hand.
- The values of education must be measured by their contribution to the most effective living.

**Scientific Education (Society-centred)**
**Main features**

- Preparation for life is its justification.
- Its favourite technique is job analysis.
- Its most awkward task is an attempt to measure the ability of students and homogenously group them in sections for instructional progress (excluding the need of young people for progress in business and society that are heterogeneous)

**Main assumptions**

- Basing the curriculum upon problems of individuals and society that are current today.
- Measuring progress and providing for skills (e.g, Shaw 1937; Hampel 2008).

**A Modern Educational Concept**

Shaw (1937: 587-589) provides a picture of this modern concept of education:

The old answer was scholarship. The new answer is that scholarship is not the most important aim of education, but personality growth rather, and social work. The old education was for the few, and it was sedentary; the new education is for all and it is active; ability to do is almost as worthy now as ability in knowing.

Shaw (1937) proposes three ways the tenets of this new theory or modern concept of education can be put into use. First, it is necessary to understand the nature of children; that while every child has specific basic needs, which are essentially the same for every other child, children also have several features which differentiate them from other children, such as differences in interests, skills, habits, capacity to learn, attitudes and appreciation. Second, the school environment contributes greatly to child development and should be comfortable, free from health hazards and strain. It should provide for the activities that are mutually interesting to students - in other words, foster a sharing experience. Other requirements are that a school should be free from fear, harsh punishment, excessive noise and excitement, undue emphasis on competition; and more important, pupil-teacher rapport should encourage creativity and spontaneity.

Third, the curriculum must be modified or changed outright. This may entail easing out traditional subjects and attempts at enrichment and preparation for vocations. Fourth, curriculum approaches that break down subject-matter and organise units of study around present-day problems or interests of the learner should be usefully followed. While this process can use more subject-matter and skills, appreciation and understanding would be achieved through the interest learners feel in pursuing their own goals.

However, the experiences through which this modern education should be delivered must be organised in some manner to indicate their contribution to development, to further learning-retention and skills, to demonstrate connection of one experience to another and to a unified whole. The role of the teacher in the teaching-learning process is to set the stage and take a back seat. There is more learning and less teaching; more activity and study and less recitation. The solutions of vital problems of individual and social life guide the pupils and learners.

Thus, this modern idea of education is a dynamic process, which involves the interplay of the educator, the learner and the social forces to make an individual socially adjustable and responsible. The modern concept of education shifts the emphasis from individual development to national development. Education is not only an instrument of social change, but it is also viewed as an investment in national development. Great educational revolutions achieve great economic evaluations.

Another idea of education that entails the interaction between the teacher, the learner and society and has much relevance for building a community of learning is Paolo Freire's theory of education, as expounded in the *Pedagogy of the Oppressed* (Freire 1974). This theory proposes pedagogy with a new relationship between teacher, student, and society. It charts the dialectic of the "oppressor" and the "oppressed" onto this relationship, referring to traditional pedagogy as the "banking model" because it treats the student as an empty vessel to be filled with knowledge. But he argues for pedagogy to deal with the learner as a co-creator of knowledge.

Assumptions of the theory that are particularly applicable to the idea of building a community of learning in community health are as follows:

- Freire argues that dialogue enables a person to overcome the limitations of ignorance and the culture of silence and then through reflection becomes more assertive in their outlook on the world.

- This transformation empowers an individual with the skills set needed to take full control of their own lives.
- Education either perpetuates the existing order or liberates people from the shackles of oppression.
- Through incessant exposure to the oppressor's denigration of their worth, the oppressed come to act and behave inferior, accepting the oppressor as superior.
- The oppressed were despised as "lazy and drunkards" in order to exploit them.
- Mere dialogue is no guarantee for liberation; instead, true and lasting freedom can only be achieved when the oppressed consciously participate "in the act of liberation".
- The one-way transmission of information from teacher to student stifles creativity and critical thinking, which serves to preserve the status quo.
- This mode of education simply turns students into zombies who sheepishly regurgitate whatever has been passed on to them without critical appraisal.
- The two stages of the banking model are identification and preparation followed by explication.
- The great drawback of the banking education is that it distorts reality to the extent that "historical conditions" are mistaken for "reality".
- The aim of liberating education is to make the people less dependent on personality cult and rely more on their own abilities to think and act constructively.
- The best form of learning is when both the teacher and the student come together to create knowledge through their shared experience of the world.
- In this learning process, there is no hierarchical authority in that the student is at once both a teacher and a learner.
- Unlike the hierarchical mode of learning that emphasises passivity and unquestioning attitude to reality, the problem-solving education fosters freedom, as opposed to subjugation, in that it examines reality, raises awareness about contemporary society with a view to bringing about progress.
- Consequently, nothing is static; instead, reality is in a constant state of flux which can be made better through conscious efforts.
- To deny people the right to freedom of expression and thought is tantamount to violence.

Community health educators can apply the oppressor/oppressed dialectics to the dichotomy of teacher, student and community that permeate most of our thinking about public participation in community health education. Freire's description of the oppressed resonates so well with how the role of community members are often seen by health officials concerning community health projects and programmes. With regard to community health education, despite the majority of health science schools developing community-oriented experiences for learners to prepare them for their role in community health practice, these experiences situated away from universities, do not sufficiently involve the community in their planning (Unverzagt et al 1998). Also, as Bickford et al (2010) reveal, in higher education, "students and even faculty are often overlooked when seeking input on learning space design. Even if brought up in the discussions, student ideas can be ignored in favour of ideas coming from people in positions of power". Freire advises encouraging participation of individuals and understanding of differences of views, etc, and urging sensitivity to those differences

Freire's theory can provide community health educators a somewhat different approach for engaging students and communities. It can serve as a roadmap for analysing and planning learning projects in community health, such as designing online cooperative and collaborative learning projects in the community, which is the subject of Chapter 11. Using this approach, the community health educator is able to look at the tensions and contradictions in the split between faculty, students and communities and how to deal with them. Nevertheless, it remains to be seen whether any of these concepts alone can provide a workable philosophy that guides the process of building a community of learning in community health. The complex changing nature of community health demands an eclectic approach to education that includes all the ideas of education discussed above in various degrees in designing curricular opportunities for learners. For example, as we have seen in outlining the assumptions of the progressive education, traditional subject-matter can be used if it relates definitely with the problem at hand. Also, for instance, a curriculum can be based upon problems of individuals and society that are topical in keeping with the ideas of scientific education.

As it will become clear in subsequent chapters, the process of building a community of learning for community health must necessarily use Freire's theory, and the scientific and modern education concepts to a greater extent than the other theories, because it aligns much more with the principles of these concepts. It is helpful to also look closely at educational ideologies in trying to construct a philosophy that suits the building of a community of learning for community health.

## Educational Ideologies

Educational ideologies describe a number of values, beliefs, understanding and sentiments that seek to explain what education is. Educational ideologies use their own combinations of concepts and metaphors that provide insight into how educational ideologies see education and which give their followers a sense of what is right and natural for children in schools. Educational ideologies constitute systems, which give meaning to the complex and diverse practical undertaking of teaching and give general guidelines towards which this undertaking can be directed. Three of the most important educational ideologies are arguably classical humanism, progressivism, and reconstructionism.

**Classical Humanism**: It is perhaps the oldest ideology and concentrates on an elite minority. It holds that "only small elite was to have the freedom to pursue enquiry and even for them only after a commitment to the value of the state has been inculcated". This ideology, which is knowledge-centred, certainly conflicts with attempts made in the 20th century democratic societies to educate all young people (Lawton 1983). As can be seen, this ideology conflicts with, for example, the modern education concept described above, which is dynamic and ought to be accessible to all. It also contradicts the concept of lifelong learning.

**Progressivism or child-centred education**: It also has a long history and represents a romantic rejection of traditional approaches to education. Instead of stressing the transmitting of a cultural heritage, what is more essential is "the need for the child to discover for himself [sic] and follow his [sic] own impulses". A curriculum with such a foundation "would be concerned not with subjects, but with experiences, topics selected by the pupils and 'discovery'" (Lawton 1983). Lawton rejects progressivism on the grounds that its view about human nature is Utopian and does not relate curriculum to knowledge or society.

Social Reconstructionism rests on the idea that education is a means of improving society (somewhat similar to the ideas of the scientific education concept described above). Skilbeck (1976) outlines Reconstructionist ideology as follows:

- The claim that education can be one of the major forces for planned change in society.
- The principle that educational processes should be distinguished from other certain processes, such as political propaganda, commercial advertising, or mass entertainment, and that the former should, if necessary, enter into conflict with the latter in pursuit of worthwhile ends or goals.
- The aspiration to make a new kind of person who would be better and more effective than the average citizen of today's society in taking an interest in core-curriculum in which prevailing social norms and practices are analysed, criticised, and reconstructed, according to rational democratic and communication values.
- Concept of learning and the acquisition of knowledge as active social processes, involving projects, and problem-solving strategies guided, but not dominated, by teachers.
- The evaluation of teachers and other members of a carefully selected and highly trained elite of educators who are designated the agents of cultural renewal.
- The relative neglect of difficulties and of countervailing forces - a characteristic feature of all kinds of Utopian thinking of which Reconstructionism is "one of the recognisable strands" (Skilbeck (1976).

The Reconstructionist curriculum emphasises social values, which Lawton (1983, p. 36) summarises as follows:

> *...in a democratic society, for example, citizenship and social cooperation; knowledge is not ignored, but a 'why' question is never far away, and knowledge for its own sake is highly questionable; knowledge is justified in terms of individual social needs... For these reasons subjects will not be taken for granted to the same extent as in a classical humanist curriculum and various patterns of 'integrated studies' or faculty structures will tend to assume more importance than subject departments...*

Thus, the ideas advanced in the following chapters will be based mainly on a democratic kind of Social Reconstructionism. Although there may be value in the other two ideologies, the social reconstructionist ideology is seen to be most useful in a democracy, because it allows for a more effective application of the principles of community health and primary health care and the building of a community of learning for community health. Classical humanism and progressivism when compared with Social Reconstructionism are far less able to stand up to an analysis of the needs of individuals and society [or cmmunities] (Lawton 1983).

However, some components of their philosophy can be used with or merged with Social Reconstructionism, as will be clear in subsequent chapters. The Reconstructionists' idea proposes that education can be used not only to favour individuals, but also to make society better. Although the classical humanism and progressivism ideologies have influenced curriculum design, neither has adequately dealt with the significant impact of culture. In the 21st century, it is imperative to recognise that curriculum development must be based on the culture of society and student-teacher relationship. This acknowledgement is consistent with the ideas of PHC that operate on education in community health.

**Educational Focus on the Community**

The basic principles and elements of primary health care (Chapter 1) comprise an ideological framework that influences the education of health professionals. To place the concepts of PHC into education, the curriculum needs to be oriented to prepare, for example, nursing graduates:

> *...with the clinical and other skills necessary for them to serve as providers of primary health care; with the epidemiological knowledge to detect and prevent disease; with the understanding of behavioural responses required in order to promote healthful lifestyles; and with the organisation and administrative ability to plan, manage and evaluate community health programmes. An inter-sector approach and involvement of the community are crucial and individual and communities should participate in decision-making on all health matters affecting them. The knowledge gained by nurses through professional training and experience must be shared with individuals, families and communities in order to generate local expertise and self-help... Students of [the health professions] need to be provided with a clear analysis of the structure and culture of the particular society they are educated to serve, (WHO 1986:18-19).*

The concepts of PHC that demand these changes in the education of healthcare professionals for the community are, as we have seen, the ideas that are integrated into the practice of community health care in homes, dispensaries, health centres and hospitals, which constitute the different levels of health care (WHO 1985), particularly in developing countries. Thus, the PHC concepts also provide the theoretical basis for the shifts in the educational focus to the community. Shifts to more community-focused education for health professionals due to the PHC concepts are already taking place in educational institutions for health professionals. Examples of the shifts are definitions of educational programmes designed to prepare health professionals for roles in the community. For instance,

Schmidt et al (1991) define a community-oriented medical curriculum as a programme whose content considers the major health problems of a country where graduates of the programmes function. This means that, firstly, the content of the programmes is not only based on the discipline that contributes to them, but also on the problems that characterise the programmes. Secondly, the particular character of the major health problems in a specific population differentiates one programme from another. Thirdly, because problems change from time to time, programmes are highly oriented to changes in the environment. Finally, the student activities in the programmes should include issues in health education and promotion, disease prevention, health research and involvement of people in improvement of their health status.

Such an education must be a process that is transformative and developmental. Within an environmental plan, such education can take place at the various levels of an individual, organisation, community and population. However, in all instances the learning is contingent on engagement and is socially constructed. Thus, the PHC concepts and principles also represent ideologies that contribute to the theoretical foundation for the change in the educational concentration from private or isolated healthcare settings to the community.

It has been suggested (e.g. Boaden et al 1999, Blair et al 2009) that there are sharp differences between developed and developing countries in the educational focus on the community that reflect the development of medicine and medical services in developed and developing countries. Information from the WHO and from developing countries indicate that there are differences of opinion in terms of style and purpose of community practice and the education of professionals for such practice. These reflect the differences between the developed and developing world in terms of context and features of health systems and healthcare education.

Whereas developing countries have for many years focused on PHC as a result of, among other things, dispersed populations, developed countries have relatively recently adopted primary health care due to increasing high costs and demand for secondary and tertiary care (Boaden et al 1999). Also, whereas healthcare education has been subjected to professional control in developed countries, in developing countries healthcare education has been reformed because of the difficulties involved in adopting Western models of healthcare provision, such as high healthcare costs. As a result, developing countries integrated health care and professional education based on the PHC approach (Boaden et al 1999). In richer countries of the world that have also embraced the PHC approach, such integration of healthcare and professional education contingent on PHC has, as in developing countries, translated well in terms of innovations like association with key stakeholders with a shared vision, multidisciplinary working, peer-assisted learning, and widely disseminated teaching technology (Blair et al 2009).

However, despite the successes that many countries have registered through PHC implementation over the past 30 years, there are at least three main challenges (Schaay et al 2008) facing PHC that countries need to address: (1) promotion of vertical programmes by development partners like the Global Fund that while providing much needed funding for priority diseases such as TB and AIDS have simultaneously promoted the selective approach of PHC through privileging vertically implemented and managed programmes (2) the influence of microeconomic forces resulting in weakening of healthcare systems due to fiscal austerity and the loss of the momentum around PHC and (3) health sector reforms that specifically concentrate on cost-effectiveness which limits the scope of PHC to a set of technical interventions and ignoring the determinants of ill health. In the constituent chapters of Part Two, we will look at how the potential opportunities and challenges of PHC can affect building a community of learning for community health in terms of the three strategic community processes of designing learning spaces, using information and communication technologies; designing pedagogy and curricula, and co-curricular activities for learning in the community.

**Summary**

This chapter has considered different educational theories and ideologies, emphasising the importance of the democratic and society-centered conceptions as they correspond more closely with the idea of building a community of learning for community health. The basic principles and elements of primary health care comprise an ideological framework that influences the education of community healthcare professionals and supports the building of a community of learning framework. The task of creating new courses of study or new patterns of educational activity for students that include these and other concepts, principles and conditions have been outlined. The following chapter considers the nature of curriculum models through which the concepts of education we have discussed can be given tangible form as curriculum proposals for building a community of learning in community health.

# 3

## *Definition of the Curriculum Question and Curriculum Models*

There are several curriculum models identifiable in the health and education literature that have been developed to advance the business of designing curricular. These curriculum models do not describe how curricula are in fact designed, rather they present different ideas on how the planning and teaching tasks should be carried out. This chapter considers the meaning of curriculum and then describes several curriculum models that are useful for building a community of learning for community health.

### Definition of the Curriculum Question

There are two contrasting interpretations of the term curriculum. Some scholars view it as the content of a particular subject area of study (Lawton 1983). This narrow definition of curriculum is often compared with the broader meaning which includes not only content, but also how and why a subject area is taught. While some view curriculum as a direct intention, a prescription, or plan (Lawton 1983), for example, a book of instructions for teachers, others view curriculum as what actually happens in schools as a consequence of teachers' activities (Lawton 1983), for example, the performance or achievement of schools.

The aim of curriculum study is to connect these two perspectives of curriculum as intention and as a reality. The major challenge of connecting intention with reality is the gap between our ideas and ambitions and the efforts at making them operative (Stenhouse 1975). In order to address issues such as content and its justification, the translation of plans, etc., one should draw on aspects of sociology, psychology, history and philosophy (Lawton 1983). It is for this reason that the term curriculum is often seen as the means by which the experience of attempting to put an educational proposal into practice is made publicly available. It involves both content and method, and, when applied broadly, it considers the problem of implementation in the institutions it is used.

This idea of a curriculum is popular due to the fact that it is more encompassing, as it includes both content and method. Hence, it is seen to be more practical in dealing with the curriculum question. It resembles the four ways of approaching curriculum theory and practice (Infed 2010): curriculum as a body of knowledge to be transmitted; curriculum as a means for realising particular ends in students, product; curriculum as a process; and curriculum as praxis. The idea of curriculum as praxis is in many ways a development of the curriculum process model (Infed 2010), but unlike the curriculum process model, it makes clear statements about the interests it serves: it makes continuous reference to collective human well-being and the freedom of the human spirit. This notion is useful when considering an approach to curriculum theory and practice in the light of Aristotle's influential classification of knowledge into three disciplines - theoretical, productive and practical (Infed 2010).

This approach, as we will see later in the following chapters, agrees with the building of a community of learning, which is the focus of this book. When applied to curriculum planning the building of a community of learning framework takes into consideration, among other things, the nature, values, development and dynamics of society and in what ways they influence learning and the learner. This makes it an appropriate model for planning education programmes for community health professionals.

## Curriculum Models

Curriculum models can be described as simplified ideas of reality in symbolic, mathematical or graphic form. Curriculum models help explain beliefs about the character of curriculum. There are many curriculum planning models in the literature that are used in health professional education. The models occur in two main categories, prescriptive and descriptive curriculum models, reflecting the two main approaches to defining the meaning of curriculum outlined above. They include:

- the subject-centred model
- the objectives model
- the outcomes-based model
- the process model
- the problem-based model
- the integrated model

Another model is the situational analysis model that is considered to be contemporary and well-constructed (Module 1: The curriculum in clinical Education 2005). Yet another model, Beattie's fourfold model (Beattie 1987), provides a useful example of how some curriculum models have incorporated both prescriptive and descriptive models in their structures, thus providing complex and multifaceted strategies to curriculum planners. These models are discussed in some detail in this chapter.

## The Subject-Centred Model

The subject-centred model (Module 1: The Curriculum in Clinical Education 2005) stresses the content of a course and allows teachers to indicate the subjects they wish to include in their courses. This prescriptive curriculum model is widely recognised as the principal feature of the traditional approach to planning education. Besides, it is the preferred approach for secondary schools and institutions

**Table 1: Advantages and Disadvantages of the Subject–Centred Model**

| ADVANTAGES | DISADVANTAGES |
|---|---|
| • It is popular with students because firstly it matches their concept of what schooling is all about and besides they are accustomed to it.<br>• Its methodical approach of learning skills suits traditional testing, which can be easily quantified and explained to funding agencies, etc.<br>• It motivates both teachers and students because of its measureable progress.<br>• It is preferred in areas where resources for staff development are not enough.<br>• It is readily handy for both teachers and students. | • Narrows students' understanding of the wider contexts of content.<br>• Focuses on each subject in an individual context, which prevents students from having a relationship between or among subjects.<br>• Stifles critical thinking and creativity because students tend to follow the teacher's perspective only without trying to form their own viewpoints.<br>• Excludes students from the hierarchical authority upon which the approach rests. |

of higher learning (Module 1: The Curriculum in Clinical Education 2005). In the same vein, it is a preferred approach for medical education (Module 1: The Curriculum in Clinical Education 2005).

For medical education, where there is need to include subjects, its use is justified and necessary as it includes critical content such as epidemiology, infectious diseases, etc. On the other hand, it places emphasis on the essential values of studying a subject instead of its non-essential outcomes. It has therefore been overused, abused and abandoned for some kind of objectives model (Module 1: The Curriculum in Clinical Education 2005). Table 1 presents advantages and disadvantages of the subject-centred model, as discussed in the literature, for example, Module 1: The Curriculum in Clinical Education (2005).

## The Objectives Model

The objectives model (Tyler 1931) is perhaps the most well-known prescriptive curriculum model. It sets out what curriculum workers should do and to answer four fundamental questions which are based on Tyler (1931). The questions are:

- What educational purposes should the school seek to attain?
- What educational experiences are likely to attain this purpose?
- How can these educational experiences be organised effectively?
- How can it be determined that these purposes are being attained?

The model demands that curriculum planners must identify their objectives, plan the content and the methods by which the objectives are to be achieved, and finally try to measure the extent to which objectives are realised (Figure 2). This task must be done in a manner in which the four elements interact to influence and possibly change the design decisions for each other's element. This model proposes that the beginning of curriculum planning must start with the objectives of the curriculum. This starts with specification of aims, which are often considered to be general statements of goals and purposes. Because aims have been regarded as too general and limited in specificity to serve as guidelines to curriculum planners, the process of curriculum planning has focused on formulation of more accurate statements of goals from the general aims which are usually called objectives. Table 2 shows advantages and disadvantages of the objectives model, as discussed in the literature, for instance, Stenhouse (1975).

**Figure 2: The Objectives Model**

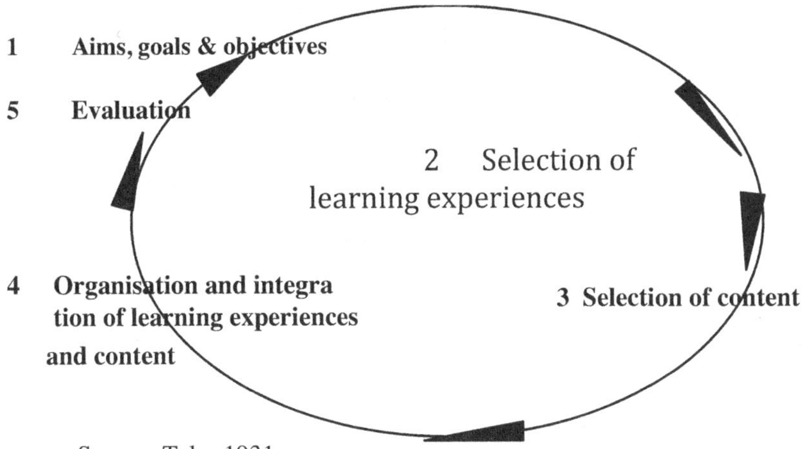

Source: Tyler 1931

**Table 2: Advantages and Disadvantages of the Objectives Model**

| ADVANTAGES | DISADVANTAGES |
|---|---|
| • It is useful in the area of training.<br>• It is appropriate in the provision of instructions. | • It places constraints on both the teachers and the pupils as it inhibits freedom of interaction that is central to the educational process.<br>• It demands the specification of objectives that are behavioural.<br>• It tries to be value-free like all scientific methods used in studying human action.<br>• It forces a hierarchical structure on curriculum planners and approaches education as an instrumental activity.<br>• Writing objectives is difficult and time-consuming, especially if as may be required each objective has to contain a statement of the 'behaviour' to be attained, the ' conditions' under which it would be demonstrated and the 'standards' by which it would be judged.<br>• It focuses on skills and knowledge acquisition only; higher order thinking skills, problem solving and values development are important educational functions that could not be written in behavioural terms.<br>• It makes the induction of knowledge difficult. |

**The Outcomes - Based Model**

The Outcomes - Based Model (OBE) (Module 1: The Curriculum in Clinical Education 2005) is a prescriptive model which proposes that curriculum should be defined by first thinking about the outcomes the planner wishes his or her students to obtain. The planner then works "backwards" to determine content, teaching and learning activities; assessment and evaluation. The use of Outcome Based Education (OBE) to underpin the curriculum process is becoming increasingly popular in health professional education (Davis 2003). OBE is often viewed as a return in another guise to the objectives model (Module 1: The Curriculum in Clinical Education 2005)

Table 3 presents advantages and disadvantages of the Outcome Based Model as discussed in the literature, for example, Davis (2003).

**Table 3: Advantages and Disadvantages of the Outcomes Based Model**

**Table 3: Advantages and Disadvantages of the Outcomes Based Model**

| ADVANTAGES | DISADVANTAGES |
|---|---|
| • Detailed descriptions of written outcomes give both teacher and student a clear picture of the competences to be attained at the end of the course.<br>• Teachers can adjust teaching methods to enhance attainment of stated objectives.<br>• Teachers can decide how objectives may be assessed.<br>• Writing lists of competences or outcomes can be useful for staff development lesson. | • Objectives may unjustifiably be given greater role in educational processes.<br>• Teaching and learning processes may become so imposed and description and voluntariness are restrained.<br>• Constructing learning outcomes and competences can be difficult and time-consuming<br>• Periodic re-appraisal of objectives and learning outcomes is an important requirement of course or curriculum development which is a continuous process. |

**The Process Model**

The process model (Stenhouse 1975) is a descriptive curriculum model that emphasises the use of principles to plan curricula and the educational process without the pre-specification of objectives. It focuses on the implementation of "worthwhile activities" that students can be involved in (Raths 1971) (Box 5). Such activities have their own built-in standards of excellence and can, therefore, be assessed. The premise of the model is that a form of knowledge has structure and it involves procedures, content and criteria. Content can be selected to exemplify the most important procedure, the key concepts, and the areas of situations in which the criteria hold.

It rests on the quality and judgment of the teacher rather than on the teacher's direction. Paradoxically, this point is also a disadvantage in that if the teacher is incompetent then the model cannot be successfully implemented. It is far more demanding on teachers and far more difficult to implement. (Stenhouse 1975).

The model is committed to teacher's personal development as it offers a higher degree of professional development (Stenhouse 1975). Among other things, it takes account of the student's individual development and needs and motivates them to integrate new content into their teaching plans.

However, Goodson et al (1975) suggest that such a list of principles of procedure and worthwhile activities might result in a definition of activities before they begin, thereby imposing the interpretation of interactions. To prevent this, they

**Box 5: List of Worthwhile Activities**

- All other things being equal, one activity is more worthwhile than another if it permits students to make informed choices in carrying out the activity and to reflect on the consequences of their choices.
- All other things being equal, one activity is more worthwhile than another if it assigns students active roles in the learning situation rather than passive ones.
- All other things being equal, one activity is more worthwhile than another if it asks students to engage in inquiry into ideas, applications of intellectual processes, or current problems, either personal or social.
- All other things being equal, one activity is more worthwhile than another if it involves reality (for example, real objects, materials and artefacts).
- All other things being equal, one activity is more worthwhile than another if completion of the activity may be accomplished successfully by students at several different levels of ability.
- All other things being equal, one activity is more worthwhile than another if it asks students to examine topics or issues that citizens in our society do not normally examine – and that are typically ignored by the major communication media in the nation.
- All other things being equal, one activity is more worthwhile than another if it involves students and faculty members in 'risk' taking - not a risk of life or limb, but a risk of success or failure.
- All other things being equal, one activity is more worthwhile than another if it requires students to rewrite, rehearse, and polish their initial efforts.
- All other things being equal, one activity is more worthwhile than another if it involves students in the application and mastery of meaningful rules, standards, or disciplines.
- All other things being equal, one activity is more worthwhile than another if it gives students a chance to share the planning, the carrying out of an activity as planned, or share the results of an activity with others.
- All other things being equal, one activity is more worthwhile than another if it is relevant to the expressed purpose of the students.

suggest trying to produce a specification to which teachers can work, thus providing the background for a new procedure to plan curricula and the educational process. To achieve this, there is need to describe the type of encounter which best characterises the new procedure through cooperative learning between teachers and students and among students. Chapter 10, which deals with pedagogical, curricular and co-curricular design presents a model of educational stages involved in learning clinical skills in the community (Boaden et al 1999) which includes a stage of cooperative learning.

As mentioned above, the idea of curriculum as praxis is in many ways a development of the process model, but unlike the process model it makes continuous reference to collective human well-being and the freedom of the human spirit. Among other things, it allows and encourages teachers and students to face the real problems of their existence and relationships, thereby confronting their own oppression (Infed 2010). Table 4 indicates advantages and disadvantages of the process model, as discussed in the literature, for example, Stenhouse (1975).

**Table 4: Advantages and Disadvantages of the Process Model**

| ADVANTAGES | DISADVANTAGES |
|---|---|
| • Emphasises active roles of teachers and learners.<br>• Emphasises certain activities because they are significant for life and in themselves.<br>• It is suitable for projects. | • Difficult to apply approach in some areas where the emphasis is on development of practical skills.<br>• It is hard to measure.<br>• Overlooks consideration of appropriate content. |

*Source:Stenhouse (1975)*

**The Integrated Model**

The integrated model (Greeves 1984) is a descriptive curriculum model that allows planners to combine separate disciplines as a whole in the curriculum. The aim of integrating curriculum elements into a conceptually meaningful structure can be achieved through this curriculum model. Such integration can be at the level of the learner as well as the content or subject matter. The learner can be assisted by organising the curriculum to analyse and apply the relationship of content, principles and concepts (Greeves 1984).

The use of the model overcomes the challenge of instruction prescribed in the form of disparate subjects. Educational impact is further increased through the provision of relevant learning experiences at the same time. The approach helps to restructure knowledge to meet changing social needs. Students receive a wider, more in-depth comprehension of academic subjects and use what they learn to real-life situations, better preparing them to succeed in whatever endeavour they choose after school.

By contrast, different subject areas may need different curriculum planning approaches, not an integrated approach. For example, a medical programme, where subjects are separate. It is also more demanding on curriculum planners and teachers in terms of time, energy and expertise (e.g. Stenhouse 1975). Table 5 presents advantages and disadvantages of the integrated model, as discussed in the literature, for example, Stenhouse (1975).

**Table 5: Advantages and Disadvantages of the Integrated Model**

| ADVANTAGES | DISADVANTAGES |
|---|---|
| • It encourages cooperation among teachers.<br>• It simplifies teachers' work as they have to deal with a few students.<br>• It provides support to traditional curriculum.<br>• It offers scheduling flexibility to teaching teams. | • Teachers can ignore the integrated curriculum.<br>• The work required to integrate subjects by teachers is time-consuming.<br>• As a result, teachers are only able to implement an integrated curriculum for only a small portion of the school year. |

**The Problem-Based Model**

A problem-based curriculum (e.g, Loepp 1999) is another type of a descriptive curriculum model. It is identified by lessons in which students are presented with a specific practical, real, or hypothetical problem, or a set of problems, to solve. Problems are defined as having no stipulated correct solution, requiring knowledge construction on the part of the students, and demanding sustained attention beyond a single lesson. Problem-Based Learning (PBL) is a pedagogical approach and curriculum design methodology often used in higher education (Loepp 1999). Box 6 shows some of the defining features of the PBL model:

**Box 6: Some defining features of the PBL model**

- Learning is driven by challenging, open-ended problems with no one "right" answer.
- Problems/cases are context-specific.
- Students work as self-directed, active investigators and problem-solvers in small collaborative groups.
- A major problem is identified and a solution is agreed upon and implemented.
- Teachers adopt the role of facilitators of learning, guiding the learning process and promoting an environment of inquiry.
- Rather than having a teacher provide facts and then testing students' ability to recall these facts through memorisation, the PBL tries to get students to apply knowledge to new situations. Students are faced with contextualised, ill-structured problems and are asked to investigate and discover meaningful solutions.

Table 6 presents advantages and disadvantages of the PBL model, as discussed in the literature, for instance, Loepp (1999).

**Table 6: Advantages and Disadvantages of the PBL Model**

| ADVANTAGES | DISADVANTAGES |
|---|---|
| • It develops critical thinking and creative skills.<br>• It improves problem-solving skills.<br>• It increases motivation.<br>• It helps students learn to transfer knowledge to new situations. | • Students cannot really know what might be important for them to learn, especially in areas which they have no prior experience. Therefore teachers, as facilitators, must be careful to assess and account for the prior knowledge that students bring to the classroom.<br>• A teacher adopting a PBL approach may not be able to cover as much material as a conventional lecture-based course.<br>• It can be very challenging to implement, as it demands a lot of planning and hard work for the teacher.<br>• It can be difficult at first for the teacher to become a facilitator, encouraging the students to ask the right questions rather than handing them solutions. |

**The Situational Analysis Model**

Using this kind of descriptive curriculum model, the planner fully considers the situation or context in which the curriculum is located (Module 1: The Curriculum in Clinical Education 2005). Curriculum developers should ask about the significant internal and external issues (Reynolds et al 1976) that will impinge on the curriculum process. Box 7 indicates the external and internal factors of the situational analysis model.

This mode of analysis is among the five important stages in the curriculum process. They are: (i) Situational analysis (ii) Goal formulation (iii) Programme building (iv) Interpretation and implementation (v) Monitoring, assessment, feedback and reconstruction. In using the situational analysis model ((Module 1: The Curriculum in Clinical Education 2005), no step should be left out and must be done systematically. But this does not mean that the steps have to be followed in a particular order.

This model is considered closer to an open-ended curriculum, because it requires the planner to consider the content of a curriculum and the external as well as the internal factors that impact on the context in which the curriculum is planned and implemented (Module 1:The Curriculum in Clinical Education 2005). Seen in this light, this model satisfies the important conception of the curriculum as a translation of educational ideas into practice. This and similar models, such as the cultural analysis model, and Beattie's Fourfold Model help us to define the essential elements of curriculum, namely situational analysis, statements of intent (aims, objectives, outcomes), content, implementation and organisational strategies, assessment, monitoring and evaluation.

**Box 7: The external and internal factors of the Situational Analysis ModeL**

| External factors | Internal factors |
|---|---|
| • Societal expectations and changes<br>• Expectations of employers<br>• Community assumptions and values<br>• Nature of subject disciplines<br>• Nature of support systems<br>• Expected flow of resources | • Students<br>• Teachers<br>• Institutional ethos and structures<br>• Existing resources<br>• Problems and shortcomings in the existing curriculum |

***Source: Reynolds et al (1976)***

However, this model might lock curriculum planners into another series of five steps which makes it difficult for them to tackle all the complexities curriculum work entails (Module 1: The Curriculum in Clinical Education 2005). Therefore, it has been suggested that though all these elements are interrelated, each essentially represents an important curriculum work open to its own investigation, debate and critique (Module 1: The Curriculum in Clinical Education 2005). But when they are taken together, they represent a comprehensive statement of the curriculum process. It must be borne in mind too that it is not easy to put all of them together and formulate simple principles for them. Table 7 presents advantages and disadvantage of the situational analysis model, as discussed in the literature, for example, Liza (2014).

**Table 7: Advantages and Disadvantage of the Situational Analysis Model**

| ADVANTAGES | DISADVANTAGE |
|---|---|
| • The model is dynamic.<br>• Its elements are seen as interactive and flexible.<br>• Its steps are conducted systematically but do not conform to a fixed starting point. | • The fact that its steps are conducted systematically but do not conform to a fixed starting point can also be seen as a weakness. |

**Beattie's Fourfold Model**

As indicated above, this model (Beattie 1987) incorporates both prescriptive and descriptive elements which are presented as four basic approaches for planning nursing curricula. These are:

- The curriculum as a map of key subjects.
- The curriculum as a schedule of basic skills.
- The curriculum as a portfolio of meaningful personal experiences.
- The curriculum as an agenda of important cultural issues.

Beattie's fourfold approach is particularly interesting as it avoids providing detailed subject –matter, stressing instead contentious issues and political predicaments in health care. Issues such as power in health care are selected because they have no particular answer and are debatable, thereby encouraging inquiry and discussion. Furthermore, the model allows curriculum planners to use complex and multiple approaches. Table 8 shows advantages and disadvantage of Beattie's Fourfold Model, as discussed in the literature, for example, Quinn (1995).

**Table 8: Advantages and Disadvantage of Beattie's Fourfold Model**

| ADVANTAGES | DISADVANTAGE |
| --- | --- |
| • Integrates the theoretical and practical aspects, thereby bridging the gap between theory and practice.<br>• Gives a sense of balance for both teachers and students, as it integrates the four design elements with teaching methods, thereby providing for the various students' learning styles. | • When the four approaches are combined, the conventional approaches tend to dominate, resulting in the student-centred ideas being included marginally. |

**The Cultural Analysis Model**

Lawton (1983) who created the cultural analysis model defines culture as the total way of life of a society and the goal of education is to "make available to the next generation what we regard as the most important aspects of culture" (Lawton, 1983, p.28). Cultural analysis, according to Lawton, is the process by which a selection is made from the culture. The cultural analysis model when applied to curriculum planning would ask these questions:

- What kind of society already exists?
- In what ways is it developing?
- How do its members appear to want it to develop?
- What kind of values and principles will be involved in deciding on Question 3 and on the educational means of achieving Question 3?

The cultural analysis approach (Figure 3) attempts to match the needs of individual youth within a specific society by carefully planning curricula. The selection from the culture is made by analysing the society that exists, how it got that way, where it is going, and then mapping out the kinds of knowledge and experience that are most appropriate. This process requires five kinds/stages of classification: (1) all the aspects that human societies have in common - the social (including health and political systems), economic, communication, rationality, technology, morality, belief and aesthetic systems - the major parameters or cultural invariants (2) the methods of analysis that can be used on a given society using the major parameters, or analysing the differences between cultures in each of the systems-cultural variables (3) classifying the educationally desirable knowledge and experiences - selection from culture (curriculum coverage), (4) consideration of the psychological theories and questions that are crucial for any curriculum development (this stage does not continue directly from the previous stages) and (5) planning of the curriculum on the basis of the cultural analysis undertaken in the preceding stages taking into consideration the psychological theories and questions that operate on teaching and learning – curriculum organisation.

**Figure 3: Cultural Analysis Curriculum Planning Model**

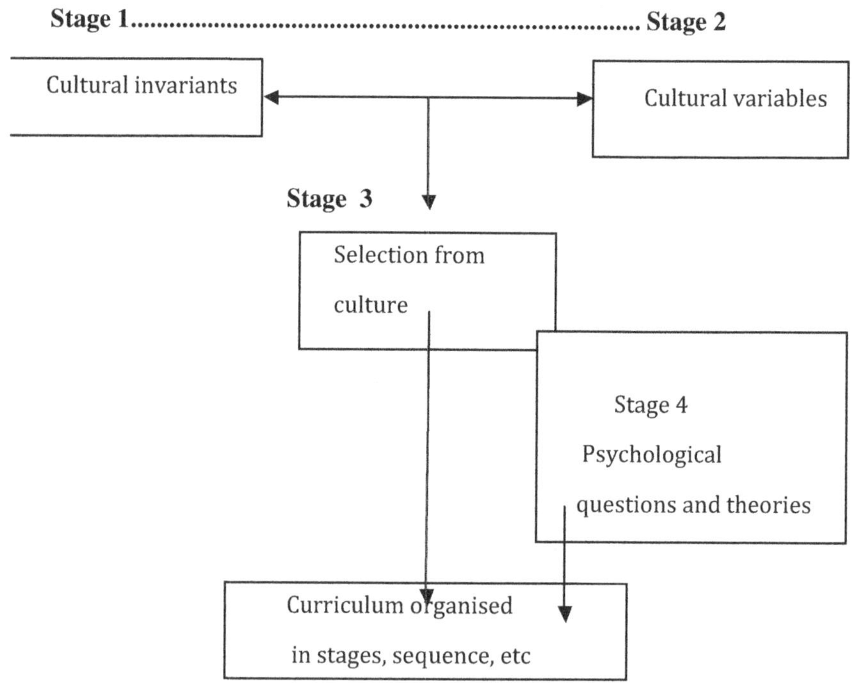


*Adapted from Lawton (1983)*

Table 9 shows advantages and disadvantage of the cultural analysis model, as discussed in the literature, for instance, Quinn (1995).

**Table 9: Advantages and Disadvantage of the Cultural Analysis Model**

| ADVANTAGES | DISADVANTAGE |
|---|---|
| • Helps to develop the full extent of possible curriculum space<br>• Indicates what may be missed by over specialisation in curriculum planning | • Seen as attempting to apply a rational system of analysis to the problem of curriculum content |

**Critique and Merits of the Curriculum Models**

The objectives model (and similar prescriptive curriculum models we have looked at) is deemed insufficient for meeting these educational requirements of community health education because they are philosophically and psychologically not that practical and humanistic for such education. The model can only be used for particular kinds of low-level skills and not the entire community-oriented curriculum. The objective model is that of a closed system, whereas in a democratic society individuals need to be autonomous through an open-ended curriculum, which is the hallmark of the descriptive curriculum models outlined above. However, such descriptive models that are more comprehensive and open-ended can be employed together with objectives (used in a restricted way) to provide a complex and multifaceted approach to curriculum planning that is much preferred to single model strategies.

An effort to solve the problem of objectives came as a proposal that each aspect of the curriculum should be examined separately on the premise that various curricular activities or subject areas will need different curriculum planning approaches. As a result of this, certain writers (e.g. Stenhouse 1975) have proposed a different type of separation of curricular activities that can be justified educationally from those that are instrumental, kinds of training for which statements of intent are not only acceptable but even necessary. This eclectic approach is a proper and acceptable approach to planning a curriculum for community health professional that fosters a community of learning.

The advantages and disadvantages of the models outlined above, such as the subject-centred, objectives and process models can apply to Beattie's fourfold model as it includes the features of these models in its framework. However, there are two shortcomings of the models that have been suggested by Quinn (1995) that must be looked at. One shortcoming is that all the models, with the exception of Beattie's model, have all been formulated for the education of children; that the educational ideologies on which they are based are tenets of childhood education. Another imperfection suggested by Quinn is the failure of all the models, including Beattie's model, to consider the requirements and opinions of service managers/employers on the outputs they need from education and training to meet their service contracts. However, as can be seen, a significant external issue in the situational analysis model that curriculum planners should ask about is expectations of employers. Some of these issues are addressed further in Chapter 10 on pedagogical, curricular and co-curricular design.

## Summary

This chapter has considered the meaning of curriculum in addition to describing several curriculum models that are useful for building a community of learning in community health. The objectives model and similar prescriptive models have been examined and considered inadequate, because they are impractical in relation to, among other things, the cultural values and behaviour and norms of a community. These models can only be applied to certain kinds of low-level skills and not the entire educational process, whereas in a democratic society individuals need to be autonomous through an open-ended curriculum. This is what descriptive curriculum models, such as the process model and cultural analysis model, are all about. Chapter 10 on pedagogical, curricular and co-curricular design explains how the models apply to the community health context on which the book is based. In the following chapter, we will examine some other theories, concepts and principles related to learning in a community.

# 4

## *Learning Theories, Process and Community*

This chapter focuses on learning theories that can contribute to developing the notion of a community of learning. Firstly, the chapter outlines several useful learning theories from education and health literature. It then considers the learning process within community settings underpinned by the learning theories outlined therein.

### Learning Theories

There are many theories that purport to explain how people learn. Each theory relates to various components of the learning process. Several of the theories, for example, Skinner (1953) and McClelland (1978) relate to trainees' motivation as well. Other theories, for instance, Gagne et al (1991) and Bandura (1986) relate to processes of learning, such as processes that occur when learners learn, retain and retrieve training content and respond to messages, and the environment in which learning takes place. This section deals with theories that have much relevance for building a community of learning for community health. The main features and suggestions of each theory are outlined briefly:

### Social Learning Theory (Bandura 1976)

#### Main Features

- People learn by observing other persons whom they see as knowledgeable and credible - behaviour that is rewarded or reinforced is likely to be repeated.
- Learning new behaviour or skills results from (a) the process of observing others and seeing the outcome of their behaviour or (b) directly experiencing the results of using behaviour or skills.
- Learning is influenced by a person's judgment about whether she or he can learn skills and knowledge.

#### Main Suggestions

- Persons cannot learn by observations unless they are aware of the important aspects of a model's performance. This is influenced by features of the learner and the model.

- Learners must remember the behaviour and skills that they observe.
- Learners should try out the observed behaviour to see if they result in the same reinforcement that the model received.
- Learners are more likely to adopt model behaviour if it results in a positive outcome.

Table 10 presents advantages and disadvantages of the social learning theory, as discussed in the literature, for example, Weeby.com (2011).

**Table 10: Advantages and Disadvantages of Social Learning Theory**

| ADVANTAGES | DISADVANTAGES |
|---|---|
| • It deals with inconsistencies in behaviour.<br>• It is optimistic.<br>• Gives a framework for integrating cognitive and social theories.<br>• Allows and accounts for cognitive processes.<br>• Explains a large number of behaviour.<br>• Easy and accurate to comprehend. | • It places lot of emphasis on what happens, not on what the observer does with what happens.<br>• Neglects physical and mental changes.<br>• Does not cover all behaviour and behavioural differences in its explanation.<br>• Fails to consider that "reward" and "punishment" may be seen differently by different people. |

Community health teachers can contribute immensely towards creating healthy learning communities by using their good position to act as positive role models for students, parents and the community. Teachers' demonstration of healthy habits such as healthy eating and regular physical activity can have a good influence on the health of students and others.

Positive modelling by administrators and teachers in community health schools can be an important step in support of such policies and actions, because it helps show real leadership and commitment students, parents and others can see.

Frequently, students watch their teachers to see how active they are, what they eat, and how they express their feelings. They can add healthy habits to many types of positive behaviour they are probably already modelling, such as modelling healthy eating habits and being physically active.

Box 8 presents a few tips that can help community health teachers achieve their "healthy habit" goals by setting small goals first (Government of Alberta 2014). Community health educators can apply Bandura's social learning theory by observing the following principles (Kearsley (1994c) :

1. Individuals are more likely to adopt a modelled behaviour if the model is similar to the observer and has admired status and the behaviour has functional value.

**Box 8: Tips on achieving "healthy habit" goals**

To help you achieve your "healthy habit" goals, set small goals first. As you experience success in meeting early goals, you can then set new goals!
Here are some simple tips to get you going:

**Healthy Eating**

- o Eat more fruits and vegetables at snack time.
- o Bring healthy foods for lunch.
- o Offer healthy food options at staff meetings and parent council meetings.

- **Positive Social Environments**
  - o "Choose your mood" each day; aim to recognise your different moods and choose to improve your outlook or attitude, or how you express your self, when necessary.
  - o Always welcome students to your class with a smile

- **Physical Activity**
  - o Get you and your co-workers moving! Consider having a boot-camp; organise a yoga or physical fitness class for staff, at a convenient time; or start a staff activity, such as a running group or volleyball team.
  - o Aim to go for a walk (indoors or outdoors) during part of your lunch hour; try to do these two or three times a week, for starters. Invite others to come along!

***Source: Government of Alberta (2014)***

2. Individuals are more likely to adopt a modelled behaviour if it results in outcomes they value.
3. Coding modelled behaviour into words, labels, or images results in better retention than simply observing.
4. The highest level of observational learning is achieved by first organising and rehearsing the modelled behaviour symbolically and then enacting it overtly.

Mentoring, apprenticeship, on the job training, and internships ( which are highlighted in especially Chapters 12 and 13 on professional development in community health and development of teaching and learning centres in community health, respectively), are strategies that agree with social learning theory (Ross-Gordon, as cited by Kearsley 1994c). Each entails learning in a social environment whereby novice learners model more experienced teachers (or coworkers) as suggested by the above example of social learning.

**Adult Learning Theory (Andragogy) (Knowles 1990)**

**Main Features**

- Adults have a need to be self-directed.

- Adults have the need to know why they are learning something.
- Adults are motivated to learn by intrinsic as well as extrinsic factors.
- Adults enter into a learning experience with a problem-centred approach to learning.
- Adults bring more work-related experiences into the learning environment.

**Main suggestions**

- Mutual planning and collaboration in instruction.
- Use learner's experience as a basis for application and example.
- Develop instruction as the basis of learner's competence and interest.
- Apply content immediately.
- Problem-centred instead of subject-centred approach to learning.

Adult learning theory was based on a need for a particular theory of how adults learn. The majority of theorists in education as well as formal educational institutions were created to educate children and youth. Thus, the art and science of teaching children, pedagogy, was the most influential education theory. This framework provides the teacher with the principal responsibility of deciding on content of learning, learning method and evaluation. Generally, students are perceived as being passive recipients of direction and content, and coming with little experience that can be a useful resource to the teaching and learning environment. Androgogy, the theory of adult learning, was developed as a reaction to such shortcomings of formal education theories. Table 11 shows advantages and disadvantages of the adult learning theory, as discussed in the literature, for instance, Conlan et al (2003).

**Table 11: Advantages and Disadvantages of the Adult Learning Theory**

| ADVANTAGES | DISADVANTAGES |
|---|---|
| • It is self-directed and allows the learner to take control of his/her learning<br>• It is broad-based and can be implemented in a variety of educational situations | • Its principles can also be applied to other kinds of learning<br>• It has been referred to in various ways, such as a theory of adult education and is difficult to classify |

Adult learning theory is particularly relevant to the notion of building a community of learning in community health. As will be seen, Chapter 12 on professional development in community health and Chapter 13 dealing with development of teaching and learning centres in community health, in particular, consider developing training programmes in community health whose audience have a tendency to be adults, most of whom had little or no formal education. A common theme in the discussion in these chapters that is consistent with applications of the adult learning theory is mutuality (1998) – both learner and instructor are engrossed in originating the learning experience and ensuring that learning happens.

**Reinforcement Theory (Skinner 1953)**

**Main Features**

- People are motivated to perform or avoid certain behaviour due to past results that came from such behaviour.
- Positive reinforcement is a pleasing outcome that results from behaviour.
- Negative reinforcement is the removal of an unpleasant outcome.
- Punishment is giving an unpleasant outcome following behaviour, resulting in a decrease in that behaviour.

**Main Suggestions**

- For learners to acquire knowledge, modify skills, or change behaviour, the trainer should identify the outcomes the learner considers most positive (or negative).
- Then trainers should connect the identified outcomes to learners receiving knowledge.
- The effectiveness of learning depends on the pattern or schedule for providing these benefits or reinforcements.
- Reinforcement theory is the primary basis for behaviour modification as a training method.

Table 12 indicates advantages and disadvantages of the reinforcement theory, as discussed in the literature, for example, Rasheed (2012).

**Table 12: Advantages and Disadvantages of the Reinforcement Theory**

| ADVANTAGES | DISADVANTAGES |
|---|---|
| • It offers a strong tool for analysing and controlling behaviour of the learner quickly.<br>• The learner conforms to the environment quickly. This is because after the learner has done the same work repeatedly and sustains it, he is given motivational reinforcement.<br>• It allows for measurement of behaviour by tests to see if the student can give answers correctly. | • The outcomes of learning may not be true because of the internal reasoning of the learner.<br>• The learner can easily conform to a poor environment that is not suitable for learning.<br>• The same set of tests that the learner goes through to ensure the learning can result in guessing of the correct answer in the final test. |

Behaviour modification is a training method that fundamentally rests on the reinforcement theory (Noe 1998). The relevance of modifying student, faculty, staff and community behaviour to enhance a community of learning in community health cannot be overemphasised. For example, in community health education many of the institutions are engaged in education that promotes learning in a community, such as interdisciplinary learning. This is accompanied by implementing new educational approaches without much attention to the possible need for modification of existing management strategies and structures. In other instances, alternative semi-autonomous organisational arrangements were set up by the established schools. Although many educational institutions for health professionals have undoubtedly tried to improve this situation by adopting existing relevant organisational arrangements or devising new ones, on the basis of the differing ideas on education, the result has still been a proliferation of many different and sometimes conflicting managerial arrangements in educational institutions and clinical settings (Kahssay 1998). With regard to interdisciplinary education, for example, there are numerous efforts to accomplish more effective interdisciplinary programmes providing experiences relevant to work in a health team. Thus model health centres for the delivery of health care have been established and are used for training different categories of health personnel simultaneously. In other programmes, courses have been developed to be taken by students of different health professions, or programmes have selected core or common–entry curricula across disciplines. Other programmes have attempted to create organisational structures conducive to cooperation. Some have added courses that make application of theory and discussion of patient care in a multi-disciplinary setting possible. Still other programmes have stressed community-based learning and problem-based learning (Stephenson et al 2002).

However, apart from the differing approaches to such education, health centres where interdisciplinary education is provided, for instance, have been generally sidelined by vertical programmes despite their critical position of delivering and linking a variety of services for the benefit of people's health and education. Despite the Alma-Ata Declaration, and even sometimes in opposition to it, vertical programmes have continued, and indeed flourished. Paradoxically, the most debilitating aspect of these programmes for health development is that they are solution-based. They emphasise targets to be reached instead of building up systems that have the capacity to promote health and solve health problems (Kahssay 1998), as well as facilitate learning in a community.

Utilisation of the small-group in backgrounds like the clinics as a learning setting is an educationally justifiable strategy. For one thing, students can be gently, but firmly, imbued with the attitude that it is desirable and enjoyable to learn and work harmoniously in groups with other pupils. As a result, classes can be remarkably self-organising, which makes teachers' workloads far less onerous than they might otherwise be. Moreover, the small-group strategy has the advantage of creating possibilities for students to learn the values and skills of inter-working with other members of the multidisciplinary health team. However, quite often health professionals in many countries justify working alone in clinical settings on the basis of ease and speed. Furthermore, the interdisciplinary and interpersonal tension that may result from co-operating with others in a team is often a reason for lack of collaboration. In addition, the hierarchical relationships and specialisation which traditional clinical care still fosters are important constraints to collaboration (Stephenson et al 2002). For example, several barriers to team work and interdisciplinary education have been reported by Wolf (1999). She also presents predictors for teamwork and concern for patients including orientation towards group problem-solving confidence, and a positive self-efficacy towards group processes. Although respect for colleagues exists among health care providers, this has been inadequate to avoid self-defeating rivalries that have constrained improvements in health professional education. Today, students who are increasingly connected devote less and less time to structured, instruction-driven learning. It is therefore proper for community health educators to look at how behaviour that constrains cooperation and collaboration can be modified as a way to improve student, faculty, staff and community engagement that fosters learning in community health. What is required in the 21st century and beyond are arrangements for learning that promotes interactions rather than boundaries or distance (Bickford et al 2010).

Chapter 11 on designing online cooperative and collaborative learning projects in community health includes steps that community health educators can follow to effectively implement cooperative and collaborative learning in the community, including a stage in which teachers should teach students to work collaboratively. At this stage, teachers are advised to look for steps in preparing their students for group collaboration in useful resources like the Internet. Box 9 presents tips (University of the Sciences in Philadelphia 2014) on how to enhance student participation and active learning that demonstrates several useful behaviour modification teaching techniques with much relevance to fostering a community of learning.

### Box 9 : Tips on how to enhance student participation and active learning

**Getting your students to work better in groups or teams**

If you require your students to work in groups or teams, you probably want them all to work effectively. Yet you probably do not have much time to devote to the topic of group performance. One way for students to learn how to function better in small groups is to give them a short article about group functioning, and have them write a short reflection on the article and how it relates to their group functioning in your course. Barbara Oakley, Richard Felder, Rebecca Brent and Imad Elhajj have found that superficial and sloppy reflection essays are predictors of problem team members. A good article for students to read is by Barbara Oakley, "Coping with Hitchhikers and Couch Potatoes on Teams" also in the Journal of Student Centered Learning 2004.

**Helping people work in groups who feel they always do all the work in groups**

Many hard-working students do not like working in groups because they feel they do all of the work, while others take advantage of them and they all get the same good grade. Their feelings may be justified. Here is a way to help these students learn to negotiate, trust and share with others.

At the beginning of the semester, before you assign students to groups, ask the students to complete the following 1 item survey and list their name.

Think about your experience working in groups. Please select only one alternative that best describes your experience.

1. I enjoy working in groups because we understand the material better, produce better products or perform better.
2. I question the value of group work for me, because I end up doing more than my fair share of the work.
3. I have little or no experience working in groups.
4. None of the above three choices fits my experience (please describe).

When you form the groups, place all the students who selected #2 in the same group or groups. These hard working students finally are in good company and can achieve wonderful things. The other students also benefit because they must learn to work harder without the one who is willing to do all of the work. The idea comes from Byrnes, JF and Byrnes, MA. (May 2007). I Hate Groups! The Teaching Professor, 21(5):8.

**Getting all members of a student group to be effective team members**

Students often complain that one person does not participate on team projects. To avoid hearing this towards the end of the semester, be proactive about the problem early in the semester. Talk about group participation; ask groups to develop rules for participation that they sign. Tell your class that they need to address team problems as they come up. If they need help in resolving conflicts, they should ask you for help. Tell students that if they cannot participate in their groups and do their assigned role, you can remove them from the group and expect them to do all of the work individually. All of these efforts are worthwhile because students can benefit so much from working on effective groups.

**Getting students to buy in and do collaborative assignments**

Students often resent collaborative assignments for many reasons. This is especially true of older, part-time or online students. Here are some ways to help students engage with and learn from collaborative assignments:

1. Explain the importance of learning to work in groups, as it will be true of most of what they do in their careers. It will improve communication skills and lead to a more meaningful learning experience.
2. Encourage students to work asynchronously using electronic tools. When students learn how to use these tools, they are obtaining a new skill that will put them at an advantage such as video chats like Tokbox (http://www.tokbox.com), ways to share presentation, work documents, etc. like SlideShare (http://slideshare.com) or Google docs (http://doc.google.com).
3. Count the process of collaborating together and not just the final grade. Assess group participation through peer assessment.
4. Make the product they produce something that really matters and is authentic. It might be a website the students can put up or a resource

guide that others might use. The added incentive that it is authentic and can be used in the real world and not just will be seen by the instructor adds much value to the assignment and its being taken more seriously.

*These ideas came from the online webinar given by B. Jean Mandernach*

**Giving a consistent message about the importance of collaboration**

One of the most important skills that employers look for is the ability of employees to work together. We often implement collaborative projects for our students. Yet in other ways we are inconsistent. If we grade on a cure especially for the final course grade, we are sending the message that only some people can really excel and some people need to fail. It is hard to get students to work together and help each other if they are graded on a complete-tive grading scale.

Karl Smith, the distinguished professor of engineering education and leader of pedagogies of engagement workshops worldwide, gave me this thought.

**Making student groups more effective**

Many faculty use student groups to engage in collaborative, problem-solving activities. Some faculty have tried them and do not like them, often because they hear from the most dysfunctional groups and not from the better functioning groups. A survey of perceptions of effectiveness of student groups found that the faculty had a much lower appraisal of how effective student groups are than the students themselves. Students reported that groups effectively resolved conflicts and saw the group activities as effective learning tools.

The best group activities involve problems or scenarios that have no right answer, require the discussion of multiple perspectives and true collaboration to solve. Students should also have enough resources available to them to complete the assignment successfully. These resources may be experts, electronic or print information, etc.

*(Citation for the study: Chapman, Meuter, Toy, Wright (2010) Journal of Marketing Education, 32:39-49)*

**Helping students to realise that they learn outside of traditional venues such as lectures**

Many of our students are so used to being taught the content through lectures, that they may not realise that they are also learning on other venues, such as more active learning through discussions, constructing concept maps of the material, or service learning. The students may see these activities as a diversion from lecturing. It may help to ask the students to reflect on their learning, record what they learned and how much they learned in these situations when they have to construct their own knowledge. It also helps if the content covered in these ways appears on tests to reinforce that this is valued content also.

*Source: University of the Sciences in Philadelphia (2014)*

However, it has been suggested that the traditional Skinnerian pedagogical approach to education is not the most effective method for teaching technology-based education (e.g., Boettcher 1998) and therefore not a very essential framework for designing ICT-supported cooperative and collaborative learning for community health. This issue is further discussed in Chapter 5 on technology, community, information exchange and learning.

**Needs Theory** (McClelland 1978)

**Main Features**

- It explains the value that a person puts on specific outcomes.
- A need motivates a person to behave in a way to satisfy a deficiency that a person is experiencing from time to time.
- These needs include the need to interact with other persons, psychological needs, self-esteem and self-actualisation needs, needs for achievement, needs for power and needs for affiliation.

**Main Suggestions**

- To motivate learners, trainers should identify trainees' needs and communicate how training programme content relates to fulfilling these needs.
- Trainees are unlikely to be motivated to learn if specific fundamental needs of trainees, such as physiological and safety needs are not met.

Table 13 presents advantages and disadvantages of the needs theory, as discussed in the literature, for example, 123 HelpMe.Com (2014).

As the needs theory suggests, to motivate learners trainers should identify trainees' needs and communicate how training programme content relates to fulfilling these needs. Also, according to the theory, trainees are unlikely to be motivated to

**Table 13: Advantages and Disadvantages of the Needs Theory**

| ADVANTAGES | DISADVANTAGES |
|---|---|
| • Gives a clear picture of the organisation so that managers know the kind of job that is suitable for an employee and the kind of workers who can further the advancement of the organisation.<br>• Gives managers an understanding on how to deal with various kinds of employees. | • A manager may make exceptions to the organisation's role in responding to an employee's needs whereby the manager violates the organisation's principle of fairness.<br>• It has little use in the public sector where employees are motivated by job security and stability, worthwhile service to society and team work, while avoiding monetary rewards, prestige and the wish for autonomy and challenge. |

learn if specific fundamental needs of trainees, such as physiological and safety needs are not met. Let us, for example, think of a community health field experience for adult learners in a rural community. No doubt this experience will not lead to learning if the learners are afraid that their job is unsecure due to a strategy to lay off workers. It is for such a reason that the policy frameworks on health inequalities which we discussed in Part One, Chapter 1 focus on the needs of health workers. For example, among the key messages of the Marmot Report (UCL Institute of Health Equity 2010) on actions required to reduce health inequalities are six policy objectives that include creating fair employment and good work for all.

There is another meaning of the needs theory discussed in Chapter 12 on professional development in community health that is connected to the need for giving professional staff the choice of suitable continuing education programmes to attend. As described in the chapter, there are centres that focus on developing the skills of facilitators and teachers from the new subject areas involved in community-based practice of their knowledge of the health service through research and consultancy which can inform their education and training roles and make them convey confidence and respect. But the character of such centres is limited in scope and at times provides a model of provision which is expensive and cannot be easily used by practitioners who require the service they provide. As Boaden et al (1999) suggest, community-based practice needs a different approach that involves distance learning that allows practitioners to attend periodically local facilities to give the needed contact which is often not possible with formal courses, access to educational material organised in a way that facilities use and offering of short courses of study.

**Expectancy Theory** (Vroom 1964)

**Main Features**

A person's behaviour is based on (1) beliefs concerning the link between trying to perform behaviour and actually performing well (2) a belief that performing a particular behaviour is linked to a specific outcome and (3) the value that a person puts on an outcome.

**Main Suggestions**

- Learning is most likely to occur when learners believe they can learn the content of the programme.
- Learning is linked to outcomes such as better job performance, or peer recognition.
- Learners value these outcomes.

Table 14 gives advantages and disadvantages of the expectancy theory, as discussed in the literature, for instance, Management Study Guide (2013).

The expectancy theory applies so well to people learning in the complex, ever-changing, and often demanding community health contexts. The expectancy theory proposes that such learning is most likely to happen when learners believe they

**Table 14: Advantages and Disadvantages of the Expectancy Theory**

| ADVANTAGES | DISADVANTAGES |
|---|---|
| • It is practical, simple and easy to apply.<br>• It can be translated into five simple steps that can help managers motivate their employees: defining the expectation, making the work useful, making the work feasible, giving regular feedback and rewarding workers who meet the expectation.<br>• It indicates the attainment factors, such as the intrinsic and extrinsic rewards felt by the worker, which drives the individual to perform better. | .• There may not be a perfect relationship between effort and performance because it is limited by one's skills and knowledge, as well as by the difficulty of the task.<br>• The specification of an outcome from some choice of job behaviour is more complex and open-ended - one outcome may lead to another in an extended sequence. For example, choosing to work hard may be associated with an increase in wages, a demand that managers may find hard to cope with. |

can learn the content of the programme (expectancy). Furthermore, such learning is connected to outcomes like recognition by peers, better job performance, increase in salary (instrumentality), and learners valuing these outcomes (valence) (Noe 1998).

**Information Processing Theory**
***(Gagne et al, 1991, as cited by Howell et al 1991)***

**Main Features**

- It gives more stress to the processes that occur when learners learn, retain and retrieve training content, and respond to messages.
- It highlights how external events, such as informing the learner of the objectives to establish an expectation influence learning.

**Main Suggestion**

- Information or messages taken in by the learner undergo many transformations in the brain.

The information processing theory's emphasis on how external factors influences learning ( apart from highlighting the processes that occur when learners learn, retain and retrieve training content, and respond to messages) is pertinent to planning ICT-supported cooperative and collaborative learning in community health. This is because community health educators need to consider such external occurrences in designing such learning experiences for students in the community.

Table 15 indicates advantages and disadvantage of the information processing theory, as discussed in the literature, for example, Mcleod (2008).

**Table 15: Advantages and Disadvantage of the Information Processing Theory**

| ADVANTAGES | DISADVANTAGE |
|---|---|
| • It acknowledges that people think - and this matters.<br>• It is a valuable explanation of learning.<br>• It is accurate and intuitive as it draws meaningful parallels to the current technologies around. | • People are not computers, but the theory makes one think we are. |

Box 10 presents several of such external events that, for example, Chapter 11 on designing online cooperative and collaborative learning projects in community health describes in more detail.

**Box 10: External events that influence learning**

- Changes in the intensity or frequency of the stimulus that affect attention.
- Informing the learner of the objectives to establish an expectation.
- Enhancing perceptual features of the material (stimulus) draws the attention of the learner to certain features.
- Verbal instructions, pictures, diagrams, and maps suggest ways to code the training content so that it can be stored in memory.
- Meaningful learning context (examples, problems) creates cues that facilitate coding.
- Demonstration or verbal instructions help organise the learner's response as well as facilitate the selection of the correct response.

**Goal-Setting Theory** (Locke et al 1979)

**Main Features**

- It assumes that behaviour results from a person's conscious intentions and goals.
- Goals influence behaviour by directing attention and energy, sustaining effort over time and motivating the person to develop strategies for goal attainment.
- Goals lead to high performance only if people are committed to them.

**Main Suggestion**

- Learning can be facilitated by providing trainees with particular challenging objectives and goals.

Table 16 indicates advantages and disadvantages of the goal-setting theory, as discussed in the literature, for instance, Management Study Guide (2013).

**Table 16: Advantages and Disadvantages of Goal-Setting Theory**

| ADVANTAGES | DISADVANTAGES |
|---|---|
| • Goals, as well as the task and timeframe, can be made clear to avoid waste on clarifying tasks or handling mistakes.<br>• Goals that are easily linked to the aims of the organisation can be set.<br>• Employees will be more committed to goals if they play a role in the decision-making process.<br>• Positive and negative feedback is essential for productivity. | • Goals that are not challenging and time-consuming are not good for goal setting as workers are unlikely to be motivated to do a good job on tasks they consider insignificant.<br>• Goal-setting relies on rewards in order to keep workers motivated which might not always be available to dispense. |

Chapter 11 on designing online cooperative and collaborative learning projects in community health also provides examples of how goal-setting theory influences, for instance, development of lesson plans. As outlined in the chapter, a step in the design process requires teachers and their partners to double-check the goals to make sure that the work is relevant to the students' goals. This is because at first the novelty of online work will soon lose its appeal if the students do not see a reason for continuing to learn a topic.

**Social Cognitive Theory** (Bandura 1986)

**Main Features**

- Social cognitive theory believes that learners have three factors that continuously influence their learning.
- The first factor is personal characteristics. This includes one's physical ability, such as being able to hold a pair of scissors.
- The second factor is behaviour patterns, which refer to one's knowledge of a subject as well as their attention span.
- The third factor is the social environment for learning.

**Main Suggestions**

- If, for instance, someone were unable to hold a pair of scissors correctly, then he would not be able to cut paper.
- If a person were unable to pay attention, he or she would be unable to retain all information.
- The environment provides opportunities and social support to a learner.

Table 17 presents advantages and disadvantages of the social cognitive theory, as discussed in the literature, for example, Meisslerm (2012).

**Table 17: Advantages and Disadvantages of the Social Cognitive Theory**

| ADVANTAGES | DISADVANTAGES |
|---|---|
| • There is accumulated and impressive research record on the theory<br>• It is concerned with important human behaviour<br>• It is an evolving theory that is open to change<br>• It focuses on important theoretical issues, for example, the role of reward in learning<br>• Reasonable view and concern of people with the social implications of the theory | • It is seen as not being a fully systematised, unified theory, and loosely organised<br>• There are related controversial issues, such as "Is reinforcement necessary for both learning and performance?"<br>• It neglects certain areas, such as ignoring maturation and changes over the lifespan<br>• Findings on the theory are preliminary, such as "Are cognitive processes the basic concepts of personality?" |

The social cognitive theory argues for a rich environment in which students and faculty share meaningful experiences that go beyond the one-way information flow characteristic of typical lectures in traditional classrooms. This theory stresses that people learn by observing other people whom they believe are knowledgeable and credible, and that learning is influenced by a person's judgement concerning whether he or she can successfully learn knowledge and skills.

Lin (2013), for example, compares the social cognitive theory (SCT) and the social learning theory (SLT) described above. She states that Bandura has proposed both the SLT (1976) and SCT (1986). She suggests that the SCT is more comprehensive than the SLT; that the SCT emphasizes the process of triangulate reciprocal determinism, which she says, consists of behaviour, personal factors and environment. Additionally, she proposes that "self-efficacy" (a person's judgment about whether he/she can possibly learn knowledge and skills) is the core factor in the triangulate mechanism. This perhaps makes the social cognitive theory more applicable to community/population health and PHC, and the idea of building a community of learning for community health which, as Chapter 1 in particular shows, focuses very much on environment, personal factors and behaviour.

**Minimalist Learning Theory** (Carroll 1998)

**Main Features**

- It is a framework for the design of instructions, especially training materials for computer users.

- It emphasises the necessity of building upon the learner's experience.
- The theory is associated with the social learning theory.
- The roots of the theory are identified in the constructivism education ideology outlined in Chapter 5.

**Main suggestions**
- All learning tasks should be meaningful and self-contained activities.
- Learners should be given realistic projects as quickly as possible.
- Instructions should permit self-directed reasoning and improvising by increasing the number of active learning activities.
- Training materials and activities should provide for error recognition and recovery.
- There should be a close linkage between the training and actual system.

Table 18 shows advantages and disadvantages of the minimalist learning theory, as discussed in the literature, for example, Balcom (2001).

**Table 18: Advantages and Disadvantages of the Minimalist Learning Theory**

| ADVANTAGES | DISADVANTAGES |
|---|---|
| • It has the potential to exist as a narrative theory in its own right.<br>• It provides democratic entities the ability to accommodate a wide-range of traditions and ideas.<br>• It has the ability to promote certain traits held to be democratic, such as increased participation and the protection of rights.<br>• It reminds us how easy it is to say too much when trying to give help. Speaking in generalities, working with abstractions, reading about a task can be as much an obstacle as a help to the acquisition of new skills. Staying on the point, leaving room to reflect, staying out of the way of learners' spontaneous learning strategies are some of the relevant lessons for training design and tutoring.<br>• When faced with new problems learners apply their problem-solving skills and find the correct solutions on their own. This is different from the systematic approach in which students are taught to solve problems they have previously encountered. | • The efficiency of non-directive methods of tutoring which appears to be the hallmark of the theory has been questioned.<br>• Non-directive tutoring allows only the student's work to be the centre of the tutoring session.<br>• Seen as ignoring directive tutoring in which, for instance, a sense of accomplishment and community watching one student at a time being instructed by a mentor is realised. |

The crucial notion of the minimalist learning theory is to minimise the degree to which instructional materials obstruct learning and focus instructional design on activities that support learner-directed activity and success. Carroll feels that training that is developed based on other instructional theories (e.g., Gagne) is too passive and do not use the prior knowledge of the learner or take advantage of errors as learning opportunities (Culatta 2013). Box 11 presents an example of a guided exploration approach to learning how to use a word processor based on the minimalist approach.

**Box 11: Example of a guided exploration approach to learning how to use a word processor.**

Carroll (1990), describes an example of a guided exploration approach to learning how to use a word processor. The training materials involved a set of 25 cards to replace a 94 page manual. Each card corresponded to a meaningful task, was self-contained and included error recognition/recovery information for that task. Furthermore, the information provided on the cards was not complete, step-by-step specifications but only the key ideas or hints about what to do. In an experiment that compared the use of the cards versus the manual, users learned the task in about half the time with the cards, supporting the effectiveness of the minimalist design.

*Source: Culatta (2013)*

Thus, the minimalist theory is applicable to designing ICT-supported cooperative and collaborative learning projects in community health, which is the focus of much of the discussion in the following chapters, especially Chapters 5, 9, 10 and 11. The emphasis throughout the discussion is how community health educators can use these teaching and learning approaches to foster a community of learning for community health. Community health educators who wish to apply Carroll's minimalist theory should find the following guidelines (Kearsley1994d) useful:

- Make all learning activities self-contained and independent of sequence.
- Allow learners to start immediately on meaningful tasks.
- Include error recognition and recovery activities in the instruction.
- Minimise the amount of reading and other passive forms of training by allowing users to fill in the gaps themselves.

### Constructivist Theory of Learning (Piaget 1964)

#### Main Features

- An individual faced with a given situation will mobilise a number of cognitive structures called operational designs.
- The learning of operational designs is done through two complementary processes:

**Assimilation**: the process through which the individual includes information from the environment into the cognitive structure.

**Accommodation**: the transformation of the cognitive structure of the individual in order to include new elements of experience.

**Main Suggestions**

- The student is actively involved in constructing his or her knowledge.
- Intellectual development is an internal and autonomous process, not very much sensitive to external effects especially teaching ones.
- The student can assimilate new knowledge only if he or she has the mental structures which permit him or her to do so.
- Students reason logically immediately they attain the logical functioning level despite the content of knowledge.
- The teacher provides an enabling environment for students to discover by themselves obstacles involved in learning a new concept.
- The teacher does not impose knowledge on students rather he or she helps them in building content by themselves.
- The teacher adapts to the needs of the students.
- The teacher functioning as a guide, facilitator, and adviser, defines the objectives and learning projects which will be carried out by the learners and in so doing build knowledge on their own.
- The teacher encourages student in exploring the learning environment to look for solutions to problems to be resolved.

Table 19 shows advantages and disadvantages of the constructivist learning theory, as discussed in the literature, for example, Steakley (2008).

In the constructivist approach, the learner is actively involved in building knowledge by themselves without considering the social environment of learning.

**Table 19: Advantages and disadvantages of the Constructivist Theory of Learning**

| ADVANTAGES | DISADVANTAGES |
| --- | --- |
| • Involvement of students in their own education.<br>• Relevance to real-life situations -bridges the gap between the classroom and the outside world.<br>• Corrections for past demographic injustice- making education more accessible to girls, the poor, minorities, etc.<br>• Prevention of discipline problems -students who are engaged in dialogue are less likely to create disturbances. | • Opposed by those threatened by the intellectual empowerment of women, the poor, minorities, etc.<br>• Knowledge may be fabricated and evaluated by individuals.<br>• It can dismantle science and human rights because nationalists can have the freedom to do whatever they want to their victims, just because doing so would seem right to them at any particular moment. |

This facilitated the social constructivist approach in learning which incorporated the social environment and the culture of the learner in the learning process.

**Social Constructivist Theory of Learning** (Vygotsky 1978)

**Main Features**

- Emphasises the social aspects of the learner.
- Sees the right direction of development of individuals as going from the social to the individual rather than from the individual to the social.
- Introduces other aspects, such as interactions, co-construction, co-elaboration and team spirit in learning, additional to the constructivist concepts.
- Considers learning as the product of socio-cognitive activities link to the didactic exchanges between teacher - students and students- students.

**Main Suggestions**

- The teacher has an opportunity to work in partnership with learners so they develop their proper knowledge.
- The teacher is no longer the person who knows everything but rather a guide or facilitator in the construction process by the students.
- The teacher creates his or her learning environment into small groups to ease management or form a community of learners.
- There should be scaffolding, reciprocal and guided teachings. (Scaffolding is a tentative structure put in place by the teacher to enable a student to carry out a task which he or she could not do on his or her own. Reciprocal teaching is one in which students consider the teacher as a collaborator as he or she poses questions or facilitates understanding).

Table 20 indicates advantages and disadvantage of the Social Constructivist Learning Theory, as discussed in the literature, for example, Sandhu (2013).

**Table 20: Advantages and disadvantages of the Social Constructivist Theory of Learning**

| ADVANTAGES | DISADVANTAGE |
|---|---|
| • Social constructivism promotes learning through collaboration.<br>• It helps to increase the awareness of the interactions between the individual, interpersonal and cultural historical factors that afffect learning.<br>• It helps learners to build, organise and construct their own knowledge based on what they have learnt.<br>• It promotes knowledge sharing between the teacher and learner.<br>• It facilitates cognitive growth.<br>• It promotes democratic learning environment. | • It can be difficult to apply in a new environment. |

The descriptions of the Constructivist and Social Constructivist learning theories suggest that community health educators should consider applying these theories to maximise learning outcomes in the community. As will be seen in following chapters, constructivism is the theoretical foundation of the ICT-supported cooperative and collaborative learning approach which, as already mentioned, is a major thrust of this book.

These are important learning theories that have much relevance for learning in community and the next section considers the application of the theories and other learning concepts in the community.

**Learning Process in Community Settings**

As already mentioned community means the social context of students and their environment. Learning theories, which help to explain how people learn, argue for a rich environment in which students and faculty share meaningful experiences that go beyond the one-way information flow characteristic of typical lectures in traditional classrooms (Bickford et al 2010). It also places emphasis on people learning by observing other people whom they believe are knowledgeable and credible (e.g. Bickford et al 2010). The learning process in the community environment incorporates the learning theories we considered above and includes:

- Expectancy (the mental state the learner brings to the teaching and learning process, such as motivation to learn and basic skills).
- Perception (the ability to organise the message from the environment so that it can be processed and used).
- Working storage (rehearsal and repetition of information takes place, making the coding of material for memory possible) and semantic encoding (the actual coding process of incoming memory) which are both connected to short-term memory.
- Retrieval which is necessary for using learned material, such as cognitive skills and verbal information, involves the identification of learned material in long-term memory and its utilisation to influence performance.
- Generalising is an essential component of the learning process, not only for the ability to reproduce exactly what is learned, but also the ability to adapt the learning to use in similar but identical environments.
- Gratifying means the feedback the learner gets through using learning elements. It is important because it allows the learner to adapt answer more appropriately, as well as giving information about the rewards that may be the outcome of performance (Gagne, as cited by Noe 1999).

Gagne's instructional events (outlined above) and corresponding cognitive processes can serve as the basis for designing instruction and selecting appropriate media (Gagne, Briggs & Wager, 1992, as cited by Kearsley 1994a). Community health educators may consider keeping the following principles in mind when applying the instructional events:

- Learning hierarchies define a sequence of instruction.
- Learning hierarchies define what intellectual skills are to be learned.

- Different instructions are required for different learning outcomes.

There are several suggestions of the learning process for community health education. One suggestion, which has been mentioned, is that learning in community will have an important part to play in preparing students for their work-life to come. Community-based education helps prepare graduates to live and work in a world that requires greater collaboration. This education must provide opportunities for students to apply effectively and continually the learned abilities to their work. Such transfer of learning is influenced by the factors of student characteristics, which include the student's motivation and ability that influence learning; work environment, that combines factors on the work that influence transfer of learning; and the design of the educational programme, which comprises meaningful material, feedback, learning objectives, organisation of the educational programme, and characteristics of the learning site. Transfer of learning incorporates generalisation (a student's ability to apply learned capabilities to the work problems and situations that are similar but not exactly the same as the problems and situations faced in education), and maintenance (the process of continually applying over time new skills developed in the learning process). For generalisation and maintenance to occur, students must learn and retain their capabilities in the community.

Another suggestion of the learning process is the development of a life-long learner (e.g. Noe 1999). There are three key features of life-long education: (1) lifelong education is conceived as building upon and affecting all existing educational providers, including both schools and institutions of higher education (2) it extends beyond the formal educational providers to encompass all agencies, groups and individuals involved in any kind of learning activity and (3) it is grounded on the belief that individuals are, or can become, self-directing, and that they will see the value in engaging in life-long education (Tight 1996: 36).

Another important suggestion of the learning process for community health education is communities of practice. In higher education communities in which community members are committed to communicating with one another on an ever deeper and more authentic level include communities of practice. Here, communities of practice can be seen as groups of students, faculty and community members who work together, learn from each other and develop a common understanding of how to accomplish learning in community.

There are also several suggestions of the learning process for the design of teaching:

- Students should know why they should learn. This means that students should understand the goals or objectives of the programme.
- Students need to use their own experiences as a basis for learning. This requires presentation of content using concepts; terms and experiences students are familiar with.
- Students should have opportunities for practice. This entails having learners demonstrate the learned capabilities stressed in the educational goals and training objectives.

- Students need feedback, which is information about how far students are achieving the learning goals/objectives. Feedback needs to be given promptly and should concentrate on particular behaviour.

Chapters in Part Two, particularly Chapters 12 and 13 on professional development and teaching and learning centres, respectively, further discuss these and other implications of the learning process in community health education.

**Summary**

This chapter has concentrated on learning theories that have relevance for building a community of learning for community health. Firstly, it has outlined several learning theories in the health and education literature. Secondly, it has considered the learning process in relation to learning in the community, which is a social environment involving many people. Learning is a social process that works best in a community setting, thus yielding the best use of societal resources. Also, learning in a community has an important part to play in preparing students for their work-life to come. The next chapter looks at technology, community and information exchange which has much to do with the enhancement of the learning process in the community.

# 5

## *Technology, Community, Information Exchange and Learning*

This chapter looks at theories, concepts and principles that are related to technology, community and information exchange required to build a community of learning. First, the chapter outlines the nature of technology and information exchange, highlighting the importance of using appropriate technology in information exchange for community health. It then considers the relationship between ICTs and learning, including theoretical approaches for designing technology-based courses. It describes the cooperative and collaborative learning modes, as well as the synchronous and asynchronous learning approaches that complement them. The cooperative and collaborative learning modes appear to be more describable than other learning approaches that foster the community of learning idea and can arguably enhance the process of building a community of learning for community health.

### The Nature of Technology and Information Exchange

Technology refers to the use of applied and mechanical sciences to industrial application. The kind of technology system by which people in both developed and developing countries try to control the environment consists of simple and complex technologies, and something in between these two kinds of technologies. The majority of people living in the rural areas of developing countries, for instance, engage mostly in agriculture where simple tools are used. In mainly urban and peri-urban areas, however, technology is more complex. For example, farmers use modern equipment and systems, including computers to work in fields, etc.

There has been widespread acceptance of appropriate technology in recent years which, in industrialised societies, means "technologies that are ecologically well adapted to the local environment, small in scale and sparing of such natural resources as energy" (Jequier, 1981:541). In developing countries the term appropriate technology refers to "a wide range of low-cost technologies aimed specifically at meeting the most basic needs of the world's poorest people", with particular focus on health, nutrition, food production, employment and housing (Jequier, 1981:541). Many developing countries are now striving to meet the goals of such appropriate technology.

The developing world may be falling behind when competing for resources, but with regard to technology, it has not yet started. For example, the "One Laptop One Child" project that aims to fix this is a case in point. Its goal is to create a rugged, low-cost, low-power, connected computer for children in the Third World (One-Laptop Per Child Organisation 2014). Its XO laptop is about the size of a small textbook, with built-in wireless and a screen readable in direct sunlight (for children who school outdoors). The computer is extremely durable and energy efficient. XO laptops have already been delivered to children in Afghanistan and East Africa, with additional shipments scheduled for the Palestinian Occupied Territories. This is a good example of appropriate technology use in the context of building a community of learning for community health, whose principles are consistent with those of such appropriate technology.

The growth of appropriate technology in health care has been accompanied by increasing efforts to assess their potential dangers and to compare them with their possible values. The need to base policy decisions on evaluations on health technologies is being realised in the field of health, where the main interests are issues such as safety, cost and efficacy of health technologies. The connection between the education of health professionals for community health and the use of information and communication technologies in such education is therefore a very crucial issue to discuss; this will be done also in the following chapters.

Information exchange can be taken to mean the exchange of something told or facts learned, or news, or knowledge, or data stored in or obtained from a computer. It plays a critical role in social interactions which contributes significantly to facilitate learning and improve student engagement through community. Information is similar to data, but it is much wider. Information, as we can see, is derived from data. A database is a collection of data that is related to a particular purpose. Its typical structure consists of:

- Database (large store of information for analysis)
- File (data storage entity)
- Record (smallest units of data storage)

A country's Health Information System (HIS) is made up of all the data and records about the population's health. The sources of data include civil and vital registration (recording births, deaths and causes of death), censuses and surveys, individual medical records, service records as well as financial and resource tracking information. An Integrated HIS is designed to pool together data from a range of sources, so that all information is stored in such a way that it can be easily found by users in different locations, in a form that is suited to their needs.

The characteristics of data quality include correctness, validity, reliability and completeness. All this requires that data is stored in a readable manner; it is recorded at or near the time of event; the length of time is minimised between registering data and its availability; that the information is understandable and available to authorised people when and where it is needed.

**ICTs and Learning**

ICTs refer to the collection, storage, retrieval, use and communication of information using microelectronic systems and computers. Concerning the relationship between learning and technology, as mentioned in Chapter 4, it has been suggested that the traditional Skinnerian pedagogical approach to education is not the most effective method for teaching technology-based education (e.g., Boettcher 1997) and therefore not a very essential framework for designing ICT- supported cooperative and collaborative learning for community health.

A review of the literature on technology-based learning yields several theoretical approaches for designing courses or units of instruction. For example, minimalist theory, social cognitive theory and adult learning theory, outlined in Chapter 4, provide more useful guidance for the design of a theoretical approach for the teaching - learning process in technology. The principal differences in the traditional education approach and a web-based learning approach are related to the concentration on the learner, the learning process and teaching strategies, which are addressed by the constructivist ideology (e.g., Boettcher 1997; Dooly 2008). In relation to communication, Web-enhanced courses use Web technology and services to support distribution of course materials and students having access to the resources on the Web. Making students accountable for using and sharing information learned in education with their colleagues can facilitate transfer of learning which, as we have seen, is an important component of the learning process in community. The constructivist ideology concentrates on the student constructing knowledge and being pro-active, rather than passive, in the learning process. As we have seen, in this idea, knowledge is constructed and transformed by students. The learning process is defined by what the learner does by activating already existing cognitive structures or by constructing new cognitive structures that receive new input.

Rather than the learner passively receiving knowledge from the teacher, teaching becomes a transaction between all the stakeholders (Dooly 2008). Applying this approach, the student is faced with a problem from real life and using resources and research will devise preliminary solutions to the problem. At this point, the student will collaborate by technology with peers to compare solutions. Online communication gives the students an instrument to compare solutions, which is then reaffirmed or reassessed. The collaborative nature of the Web supports the second constructivist principle, which is that learning is embedded in social interactions (Dooly 2008).

The literature (e.g. Weidner et al 2007) demonstrates that Peer-Assisted Learning (PAL) has long been recognised in theory, research, and clinical education as an educational experience in which students encounter mutual benefits as teachers and learners. This literature suggests several positive outcomes of the PAL. The primary result is that students, who are involved actively in their learning rather than passively receiving information from an instructor, will learn more readily.

PAL is a purposeful component of professional preparation programmes in fields such as nursing, occupational therapy, and physical therapy. Other positive outcomes identified by peer- learners include:

- a decreased level of stress or anxiety when working with peers compared with clinical instructors
- improved communication skills
- increased cognitive and psychomotor improvement scores
- increased confidence in clinical skills and decision making
- improved organisational skills

Positive outcomes identified by peer teachers include:

- opportunities to practise leadership and teaching skills
- opportunities to review and enhance understanding of clinical skills

**Cooperative and Collaborative Learning**

As the foregoing discussion suggests, collaborative learning requires working together towards a common goal. This kind of learning has been given different names, some of which have been mentioned above. They include cooperative learning, collective learning, peer-teaching, peer-learning, or team-learning. What these names have in common is that they all incorporate group work. But collaboration is more than cooperation; collaboration entails the whole process of learning. This may encompass modes like students teaching the teacher, students teaching one another and, of course, the teacher teaching the students, too (Dooly 2008). More significantly, it signifies that students are responsible for one another's learning as well as their own and that reaching the goal implies that students have assisted each other to understand and learn. Contrarily, the process of cooperative learning is designed to enhance the attainment of a particular goal or product by people working together in groups. Unavoidably, cooperation and collaboration seemingly overlap; however, in the cooperative mode of learning, most of what is going on in the class is still controlled by the teacher, even if the students are working in groups. On the other hand, collaborative learning is aimed at getting the students to take almost full responsibility for working together, changing and evolving together and, of course, building knowledge together. Constructivism, outlined above, is the theoretical foundation of both collaborative and cooperative learning.

Thus, the collaborative and cooperative modes of learning are arguably the most important learning strategies through which community of learning can be achieved. Using these approaches to learning in the community, students can engage in many activities to form the social interactions needed to establish and build a community of learning for community health. They can create a community in the absence of important faculty involvement. Also, by using these frameworks, faculty, as can be seen, can have a great positive impact on shaping, contributing to, and extending the learning environment of students in the community. They can coordinate and improve pedagogical approaches, the curriculum, and the co-curricular experiences of students with the goal of creating community that is learner friendly and is based on participation.

**Synchronous and Asynchronous Learning**

As we have seen, network-based learning is a good way to design tasks that include ways of giving students the chance to analyse, synthesise, and evaluate their ideas together in groups within the cooperative/collaborative modes of learning. These higher order thinking skills of analysing, synthesizing and evaluating can be learned synchronously or asynchronously. Such learning is needed in community health for tackling the factors that influence community or population health. Thus, the synchronous and asynchronous learning modes complement cooperative/collaborative learning in the educational process. Asynchronous learning is a student-centred teaching method that uses online learning resources to facilitate information sharing outside the constraints of time and place among a network of people. Asynchronous learning is based on the constructivist theory, a student-centred approach that, as already mentioned, emphasises the importance of peer-to-peer interactions. This approach combines self-study with asynchronous interactions to promote learning, and it can be used to facilitate learning in traditional on-campus education, distance education, and continuing education. This combined network of learners and electronic networks in which they communicate are referred to as an asynchronous learning network. In contrast, synchronous learning takes place when two or more people are communicating in real time. Sitting in a classroom, talking on the telephone, chatting via instant messaging are examples of synchronous communication. So is sitting in a classroom a world away from where the teacher is speaking via teleconferencing. Table 21 presents advantages and disadvantages of synchronous and asynchronous learning, as discussed in the literature, for example (Kaplan et al 2003):

**Table 21: Advantages and Disadvantages of synchronous and asynchronous learning**

| ADVANTAGES | DISADVANTAGES |
|---|---|
| **Synchronous Learning**<br>• Increases arousal, motivation, and convergence on meaning.<br>• Learners are eager to give their input on an issue.<br>• Adult learners are more stimulated intellectually when an immediate response is expected.<br>• Useful in discussing less complex issues.<br>• Gives the adult learner the ability to discuss more basic topics with short reflection time.<br>• Excellent for social interaction and discussing multiple topics in one session. | **Synchronous Learning**<br>• Time spent off subject can be significant.<br>• Learners may spend time discussing issues not relevant to the topic<br>• Can lead to distractions and a waste of time.<br>• It can be affected by personal schedules and planning. |

| ADVANTAGES | DISADVANTAGES |
|---|---|
| **Asynchronous Learning**<br>• Helpful when reflecting on complex issues since an immediate answer is not expected.<br>• Gives time to process information.<br>• Important when synchronous meetings cannot be scheduled.<br>• Most of the time is spent on subject.<br>• Time spent off subject is kept to a minimum.<br>• Improves work efficiency of time committed to tasks. | **Asynchronous Learning**<br>• Social interaction is limited to text or other non-interactive type media.<br>• Students feel distant or separated from group.<br>• Exchange of ideas is limited.<br>• I t can lead to confusion and prolonged planning of tasks. |

Part Two, Chapter 9 on technology, community, and information exchange in learning describes the ICT tools that can be used to facilitate these two learning modalities, and a section in Chapter 10 on Pedagogical, Curricular, and Co-curricular Design shows in more detail how the methods of asynchronous and synchronous learning can be used in the community.

Bickford et al (2010), for instance, outline several pedagogical and curriculum approaches to fostering a community of learning (see Part Two, Chapter 8, Table 35). These approaches interestingly include elements of cooperative/collaborative learning and the asynchronous and synchronous learning modes that are related to them. However, this book (particularly Part Two which applies the concepts and theories outlined in Part One) refers especially to the cooperative and collaborative learning forms as a means of succeeding with the task of building a community of learning for community health. There are several reasons for this. The first one is that a main aspect of the WHO's drive towards global health reform around the 1980s is a requirement for extreme changes in the nature and location of healthcare education that is consistent with several declarations (e.g. World Federation for Medical Education 1988) that called for educational activities which encourage and develop teamwork among people who will function together in particularly primary health care. The second one is that studies of best practices in education for community-oriented health professions (e.g. Edwards et al 1998) have shown that most programmes maintain an interdisciplinary approach to teaching PHC, where members of a profession work collaboratively with members of other professions. The third reason is that the cooperative and collaborative learning concepts, particularly collaborative learning, get students to build knowledge together, which enhances the student's education in community health where after graduation he/she will have to deal with the factors that influence community health. These factors, as already indicated, reflect the realities (Part One, Chapter 1) that were instrumental in the development of the PHC in the past three decades and will remain the major determinants of the health situation in the 21st century.

The fourth reason is that the cooperative and collaborative learning modes appear to be more definable than other learning modes that foster a community of learning and, therefore, better enhance understanding of educational processes that foster a community of learning.

Part of the problem, argues Smith (1996), is that community learning, for example, is used in a rather loose way and there does not appear to have been much open conceptualisation. But this statement shows that it is the role of community educators to enhance both teaching and learning techniques in the community and community of learning. Indeed, as we indicated in Part One, Chapter 3, for the curriculum process model (one of the descriptive curriculum models we consider most important for accommodating the realities of PHC) to be used most effectively in the educational process) community health educators must try to produce a specification to which teachers can work with in using the curriculum process, thereby giving the basis for a new usage. This can be accomplished by describing the type of encounter which best characterises the new usage through cooperative and collaborative learning between teacher and students and between students. Chapters in Part Two of this book concentrate on using cooperative/ collaborative teaching and learning as the principal learning modes of fostering a community of learning in community health.

**Summary**

This chapter has looked at learning theories, concepts and principles in connection with technology, community and information exchange to build a community of learning. Firstly, it has outlined the nature of technology and information exchange, highlighting the importance of using appropriate technology in information exchange for community health. Secondly, it has considered the relationship between ICTs and learning, including theoretical approaches for designing technology-based courses. It describes the cooperative and collaborative teaching and learning modes, as well as synchronously and asynchronously learning that together appear to enhance educational processes that can help build a community of learning for community health. The following chapter considers leadership and management theories that can be useful to the leader in this building process.

# 6

# *Leadership and Management Theories*

Leadership and management theories as described in the relevant literature fall into two general categories: micro–level theories and macro-level theories. Micro-level theories help explain and predict individual behaviour (e.g. motivation theories) and interpersonal issues (e.g. leadership theories, communication theories, and theories of group dynamics). Macro-level theories explain issues at a broader, agency level. These theories focus on the best ways to organise work, on how to obtain the resources necessary to accomplish agency goals, on organisational level change, and on power dynamics. The organisational-level theories that are particularly relevant for population-focused health interventions and building a community of learning in community health include structural contingency theory, institutional theory, and resource dependence theory. Managers and consultants often ask which form of organisational structure will best promote the efficient achievement of organisational goals. This chapter presents the main suggestions or assumptions of several useful examples of such theories in each category that the community health education leader and his/her team can use for building a community of learning for community health.

## 1 Micro-Level Theories
## Leadership Theories

**Orlando's Model of Nursing** (Orlando 1990)

- It offers suggestions that are especially appropriate for leadership in the community (Laurent 2000).
- It proposes that the public health nurse is functioning as a leader and partner when he or she works with community members to identify community health needs and needed policies and programmes.
- It concentrates on a partnership that includes the client in every step of decision-making about care.

Compared to other task-oriented theories, Orlando's theory strengthens the role of the nurse as an advocate for the patient. The nurse constantly revises the care process through continuous validation of his or her findings with that of the patient. This prevents the formulation of ineffective plans or improper diagnosis.

Table 22 shows advantages and disadvantages of Orlando's model of nursing, as discussed in the literature, for example, Gonzalo (2011).

**Table 22: Advantages and Disadvantages of Orlando's Model of Nursing-**

| ADVANTAGES | DISADVANTAGES |
|---|---|
| • It assures that the patient is treated as an individual and will have an active and constant input in his/her own care.<br>• It asserts nursing's independence as a profession and its belief that this independence should be based on a sound theoretical framework.<br>• It guides the nurse to evaluate his/her care in terms of objectively observable patient outcomes. | • It lacks the operational definitions of society or environment which limits the development of research hypothesis.<br>• It focuses on short-term care, not usable in long-term care.<br>• Unconscious patients are not included in the theory. |

**Contingency Leadership Theory (Fiedler 1967)**

It suggests that:

- The most effective leadership style is dependent on characteristics of the relationship between leaders and followers, the situation and task.
- The most effective leadership style rests on the degree of knowledge and maturity of group members.
- The health worker who leads should know the level of skill, maturity and motivation of the team members and adjust his/her leadership style accord ingly.
- Individuals who have technical expertise are, among other things, highly motivated (the leader in this instance operates more as a facilitator and less as a supervisor).
- Individuals who are less familiar with the task or less self-directed, on the contrarily, will be more productive when the leader concentrates on completing the task through coaching, supervising, and follow-up.

The model includes three distinct elements and two distinct styles. The elements on which a situation is assessed are:

- Good or bad member-leadership relations

- High or low task structures
- Strong or weak position power

The basis of the two distinct styles is the leader being either task-oriented or relation-oriented.

Table 23 indicates advantages and disadvantages of contingency leadership theory, as discussed in the literature, for example, Brown (2001).

**Table 23: Advantages and Disadvantages of Contingency Leadership Theory**

| ADVANTAGES | DISADVANTAGES |
|---|---|
| • In general it is good for evaluating the performance of a leader.<br>• It leads to more effective and precise leadership.<br>• It can help close relationship between workers and leaders develop more easily.<br>• It helps leaders to know the specific tasks they are responsible for without confusion. | • It does not take account of all types of jobs in existence.<br>• Determining who the leader should be based mainly on the person's ability to handle stress can lead to an erroneous situation.<br>• Its method of measuring leadership is considered inappropriate. |

The theory is especially relevant to population and community-focused health care where health workers often function independently in clients' homes or in mobile clinics or other areas where supervision may be difficult.

**Path-Goal Leadership Theory (House 1971)**

- It concentrates on individual goals and meeting individual needs.
- It declares that good leaders must first of all assist others identify their goals and then develop means to assist them achieve those goals (this way, leaders serve as facilitators who identify a path for achieving the goal and remove barriers along the path).
- It suggests that a principal goal of such a leader is helping individuals identify their educational needs and working with them to help them meet those needs.

The leader sees a path that needs to be trodden, one leading to the accomplishment of a goal and he/she attempts to clear it and get the group members to tread on it, using various techniques such as cajoling. Path-goal theory can be considered a variant of transactional leadership theory where the leader is clearly directing activity and the only factor that varies is the manner in which this is done. There are some aspects of contingency theory as well, where various means of applications vary with the situation.

Table 24 gives advantages and disadvantages of the Path-goal leadership theory, as discussed in the literature, for instance, Leadership Central. Com (2013).

**Table 24: Advantages and Disadvantages of the Path-Goal Leadership Theory**

| ADVANTAGES | DISADVANTAGES |
|---|---|
| • It contributes to our understanding of leadership through empirical tests.<br>• It is instrumental in the development of new perspectives in the leadership field.<br>• It suggests that there is need for flexibility in theory formulation.<br>• Its ideas are easy to convey. | • It is seen as being undemocratic, as it assumes that group members do not know what is good for them.<br>• If the leader has flaws the whole method stands a chance of failure.<br>• Leaders are not always rational and a course of action might be based on delusion, thereby jeopardising group members.<br>• Too much dependence on the leader might lead to collapse of the leader-led task system if, for example, the leader cannot for some reason carry out his/her leadership functions.<br>• Its measurement of leadership behaviour is considered improper. |

Different groups of people involved in building a community of learning for health have personal needs and dreams. This theory can help to extend these needs and dreams to become the common need and dream of people participating in building a community of learning for community health.

**Transformational Leadership Theory** (Burns 1978)

- Unlike contingency and path–goal theories that concentrate on identifying the best possible means to achieve a given goal, transformational leadership deals with the goal itself and the relationship of the goal to values.
- It includes the needs of both organisations and individuals.
- It suggests that:
- The leader should motivate followers to achieve a vision that matches their values (Burns, 1978; Dunham-Taylor, 2000).
- The leader should influence others to work towards achieving something new, like a new dream that has not yet been imagined.
- The leader is capable of changing the situation to one that is unlike the status quo.
- The leader is a good communicator, has inspirational traits and a trustworthy character and can promote teamwork.

Table 25 indicates advantage and disadvantages of transformational leadership, as discussed in the literature, for example, Kokemuller (2015a).

**Table 25: Advantage and Disadvantages of Transformational Leadership Theory**

| ADVANTAGE | DISADVANTAGES |
|---|---|
| • It is a leadership theory that believes that people rise higher through positive motivation than negative motivation. | • It does not include the dynamics of a situation and assumes that followers would want to work together to achieve a goal.<br>• Its approaches are not as effective in situations where followers do not have the skills or experience necessary to complete a task, or are not motivated to perform without an immediate or tangible reward.<br>• Its results take time to happen. |

Transformational leaders are sometimes found in learning organisations, or agencies that create cultures supporting ongoing learning, experimentation, and creation of new knowledge and is therefore important for building a community of learning where, as the theory suggests, there is essentially a need to promote a culture of safety and positive work environments for others. In the context of building a community of learning for community health, such learning organisations and work environments include community agencies and organisations, as well as teaching and learning centre that provide professional development opportunities (to be discussed in Part Two, Chapters 12 and 13)

**Motivational Theories**

**Maslow's Theory of Human Needs** (Maslow 1943)

- Perhaps the most well-known motivational theory (Maslow, 1970).
- Modified by Alderfer (1972) suggesting that people have only three basic needs: existence, relatedness, and growth needs; that people do not constantly strive to meet a higher-level need, as Maslow has stated, but often remain at a certain level.

Table 26 shows advantages and disadvantage of Maslow's theory of human needs, as discussed in the literature, for example, Kaur (2013).

.

Many examples related to this theory can be drawn from the health field. For example, community health workers who are working in situations such as understaffing and high–stress situations may operate at the existence level, until their situation changes.

**Table 26: Advantages and Disadvantage of Maslow's Theory of Human Needs**

| ADVANTAGES | DISADVANTAGE |
|---|---|
| • It suggests that individualism is autonomous with human rights and democracy.<br>• It suggests that individualism is built on equal treatment under the law.<br>• It helps managers to understand the behaviour of their employees.<br>• It helps managers to provide the right kind of financial and non-financial motivation for their employees. | • Employees may not want or require the need offered them or are likely to accept them. |

**Bandura's Social Learning Theory (Bandura 2001)**

- Proposes (Bandura 2001) that people learn in part from role models and that confidence in one's ability to reach a goal is a key to motivation and the ability to sustain effort to achieve goals.

Table 27 presents advantages and disadvantages of Bandura's social learning theory, as discussed in the literature, for example, Weebly (2011).

**Table 27: Advantages and Disadvantages of Bandura's Social Learning Theory**

| ADVANTAGES | DISADVANTAGES |
|---|---|
| • It deals with inconsistencies in behaviour.<br>• It is optimistic.<br>• It gives a framework for integrating cognitive and social theories.<br>• It allows and accounts for cognitive processes.<br>• It explains a large number of behaviour.<br>• It is easy and accurate to comprehend. | • It places a lot of emphasis on what happens, not on what the observer does with what happens.<br>• It neglects physical and mental changes.<br>• It does not cover all behaviour and behavioural differences in its explanation.<br>• It fails to consider that "reward" and "punishment" may be seen differently by different people. |

As mentioned in Chapter 4 where the theory is also discussed, educators functioning in the community should know that they serve as role models for colleagues and students, and sometimes for lay people in the community as well.

For example, community health educators who are particularly skilled in conflict resolution or building coalitions can help develop this skill through role modelling, goal setting, and coaching. Such good leadership skills are essential for faculty leaders working in the community.

**Locke's Goal-Setting Theory (Locke et al 1979)**

- It suggests that people are more motivated to achieve goals that they participate in setting, that are challenging, and for which they receive regular feedback.
- It is a technique used to increase incentives for workers to complete work quickly and effectively.

Table 28 indicates advantages and disadvantages of Locke's goal-setting theory, as discussed in the literature, for example, Kokemuller (2015b).

**Table 28: Advantages and Disadvantages of Locke's Goal-Setting Theory**

| ADVANTAGES | DISADVANTAGES |
|---|---|
| • Goals, as well as the tasks and timeframes can be made clear to avoid waste on clarifying tasks or handling mistakes.<br>• Goals that are easily linked to the aims of the organisation can be set.<br>• Employees will be more committed to goals if they play a role in the decision-making process.<br>• Positive and negative feedback are essential for productivity. | • Goals that are not challenging and time-consuming are not good goal- setting as workers are unlikely to be motivated to do a good job on tasks they consider to be insignificant.<br>• Goal-setting relies on rewards in order to keep workers motivated which might not always be available to dispense. |

This theory agrees well with the democratic principles of the PHC, which were outlined in Chapter 1, such as the principle of self-reliance. It is particularly relevant for building a community of learning in community health, particularly in terms of stakeholder participation, which is a subject of the following chapters.

**2. Macro-Level Theories**

**Structural Contingency Theory (Pfeffer 1982)**

- It includes organisational structure which refers to the ways people in an agency organise themselves to achieve the mission and goals of the agency. (Such organisation is aided by drawing a picture of the organisational chart, which illustrates the formal lines of authority in the agency, and written documents that define how the agency will operate. Such documents include the mission, vision, values, goals, philosophy, policies, procedures, and job descriptions).

- It includes in every agency an informal structure - the manner in which people actually work together. (This includes informal communication patterns, informal sources of power, and unwritten rules of conduct).

Table 29 gives advantages and disadvantages of the structural contingency theory, as discussed in the literature, for example, Donaldson (2006).

**Table 29: Advantages and Disadvantages of the Structural Contingency Theory**

| ADVANTAGES | DISADVANTAGES |
|---|---|
| • It stresses that the context in which people work matters when deciding how to organise the work.<br>• It posits that there is not a single superior structure that can be applied to every organisation. In order to produce high performance organisational design must consider structural factors influencing structure and create a structure that fits these situational factors or contingencies.<br>• Decentralised organisations give more authority to lower level employees, resulting in a sense of empowerment (however, some employees are more comfortable in organisations where their managers confidently give instructions and make decisions)<br>• Centralised organisations can be less costly and wasteful. | • It is static and fails to deal with organisational change and adaptation<br>• It focuses primarily on single organisation where the focus is only on one's organisation interaction with its environment, not the external environment which ultimately impacts many organisations. |

Faculty leaders working in the community should be familiar with both formal and informal agency structures. There are three conditions under which agencies can have more formal structures:

- when employees perform routine tasks that are not expected to vary a great deal
- when employees do not have high levels of professional education
- when the industry or environment in which the agency operates is stable and not changing very much

Normally, as agencies grow larger they become more highly structured, or formalised. This is often the case in large health departments, home health agencies, school districts, and healthcare clinics. Contrarily, organisations that accomplish their goals through the work of highly skilled professionals, that provide individual services that are expected to vary across clients, and that operate in a turbulent, rapidly changing environment are more likely to be successful if their structures are looser (Burns et al 1961), allowing employees latitude and autonomy in making decisions.

Presently, some community healthcare organisations are moving towards more organic structures despite sometimes being very large. Individual units, departments, or programmes often function very autonomously. This places a great deal of authority and responsibility in the hands of healthcare managers. Employees are likely to feel more empowered to do their work in a more organically structured environment that supports clinical autonomy and collaborative professional relationships. In other cases, organisational leaders choose a more centralised approach, partly because these structures tend to be less costly and wasteful, especially in resource constraint healthcare settings. A health department with only a few major clinical departments, for instance, will spend less on administrative overhead than one with numerous smaller clinical departments, each of which has its own managers and support staff. It has been suggested that this is why despite the strong push for decentralisation, not much has been achieved in implementing this important principle of PHC. Loose or organically structured organisations are more likely to be decentralised, with much decision-making authority pushed down to the lowest level in the agency where employees have the information needed for making decisions. These issues are further discussed in Part Two, particularly in Chapter 13 which discusses the development of teaching and learning centres in community health.

**Institutional Theory (Scott 1995)**

- Concentrates on how formal and informal values and norms affect agency activities.
- Suggests that agency members are more likely to respond to widely shared values and norms of behaviour than they are to formally written policies and procedures.
- The fundamental feature and principle of institutional theory is conformity. This is used for determining an organisation's legitimacy. This concept demands that an organisation incorporate particular rules, norms and requirements into its mission and goals. Also, the concept emphasises the turning points of environmental factors and their influence on organisations (Goodin 1995).

Table 30 indicates advantages and disadvantages of the institutional theory, as discussed in the literature, for example, Donaldson (2006).

**Table 30: Advantages and Disadvantages of Institutional Theory**

| ADVANTAGES | DISADVANTAGES |
|---|---|
| • It can be a rewarding concept to an organisation because society plays a vital role in determining the legitimacy of an organisation directly, and has more power in the operations of an organisation- it bridges the gap between societal views and an organisation's actions.<br>• As a result of conformity many organisations begin to resemble one another because they are faced with the same societal pressure. This can be beneficial because it can offer an alliance between organisations with the same focus. | • Places a tremendous amount of constraint on management to conform to the norms, rules or requirements of an organisation.<br>• High level of constraint can be bad for an organisation because it can inhibit visibility, creativity and diversity within a particular field.<br>• The legitimacy of an organisation like a school can be questioned if it uses, for example, a non-traditional methodology of learning.<br>• Management may have a minimal amount of freedom to make decisions which may hinder the structural process within an organisation.<br>• The concept of legitimacy often makes organisations resistant to change for fear of breaking away from the norm because their legitimacy may be challenged. |

This explains why organisational culture is important. Faculty leaders working in the community must be aware of the powerful influence that rules, values and norms play in agency work and collaborate with others to promote a culture of safety, etc. There are many examples of how the principle of conformity is encouraging or constraining efforts at providing more effective health care to communities. As discussed in Chapter 4, health centres where interdisciplinary education is provided, for instance, have been generally sidelined by vertical programmes despite their critical position of delivering and linking a variety of services for the benefit of people's health and education. Vertical programmes have continued, and indeed flourished despite the Alma-Ata Declaration, and even sometimes in opposition to it (Kahssay 1998).

**Resource Dependence Theory (Pfeffer et al 1978)**

- This is basically about power, keeping it and maintaining it. It suggests that the primary motivator for organisational behaviour is the desire to reduce uncertainty about getting the resources necessary to operate (these resources are usually financial but may also include key personnel, seats on influential community boards, or persons opposed to effort at getting the needed resources, who are with prestigious organisations). Table 31 shows advantages and disadvantages of the resource dependence theory, as discussed in the literature, for example, Nienhuser (2008).

**Table 31: Advantages and Disadvantages of Resource Dependence Theory**

| ADVANTAGES | DISADVANTAGES |
|---|---|
| • It is theoretically well confirmed.<br>• Generally, it significantly contributes to explaining behaviour, structure, stability and change of organisations.<br>• Its strategies could be used to buffer environmental pressures and reduce uncertainty. | • Its propositions about which conditions are required for organisations to fit in to the environment, to resist or to actively change their environment are not very precise.<br>• The relationship between securing resources and power has not been clarified. |

To be effective, community health faculty leaders must be able to accurately analyse power issues both within an agency and within the community. They must be able to predict the resource requirements of the agency and how managing those resources may affect power issues within the system. For the purpose of building a community of learning in community health, examples of important resources include space, budgets, staff, equipment, and community agencies and groups. Faculty leaders must try to ensure that they have adequate resources to achieve their mission, vision, and goals for building a community of teaching and learning interventions. This theory, therefore, has much significance for building a community of learning for community health where, as the chapters in Part Two show, a major part of the faculty leader's responsibility has to do with resource issues.

**Roy's Adaptation Model of Nursing (Roy et al 1999)**

- This which includes nursing management argues that agencies, such as community agencies, are made up of interdependent systems.
- It is helpful for explaining and predicting how community health faculty leaders/managers and consultants can help agencies adapt to change.
- Faculty leaders function as change agents in the community because they foster agency adaptation.
- Faculty leaders must analyse how well interdependent units function to achieve agency goals.

Table 32 presents advantages and disadvantages of Roy's adaptation model of nursing, as discussed in the literature, for example, Gonzalo (2011).

**Table 32: Advantages and Disadvantages of Roy's Adaptation Model of Nursing**

| ADVANTAGES | DISADVANTAGES |
|---|---|
| • It suggests multiple causes in a situation which is useful when dealing with multifaceted human beings.<br>• Its sequence of concepts follows logically and every concept is operationally defined.<br>• Presentation of each concept includes a recurring idea of adaptation.<br>• Its concepts are stated in relatively simple terms.<br>• Guides nurses to use observation and interviewing skills in doing an individualised assessment of each person.<br>• Its concepts are applicable within many practice settings of nursing. | • Painstaking application of the model requires significant input of time and energy.<br>• It has many elements, systems, structures and multiple concepts.<br>• It does not state how to prevent or resolve mal-adaptation. |

Systems theories are important for building a community of learning because they include parts of micro-and macro-level organisational theories and help explain the dynamics of rapid, interconnected change and the emergence of patterns of activity. These issues are also further considered in the chapters of Part Two, particularly Chapters 12 and 13 which discuss professional development and teaching and learning centres respectively.

**Complex Adaptive Systems Theory (Mitleton-Kelly 1997)**

- It suggests that combining unpredictability and interdependence leads to disequilibrium and possibility to adaptive systems.
- Basic features of complex adaptive systems are autonomous agents, network structures, and profuse experimentation.

Table 33 shows advantages and disadvantages of the complex adaptive systems theory, as discussed in the literature, for example, The Health Foundation Inspiring Improvement (2010).

**Table 33: Advantages and Disadvantages of Complex Adaptive Systems Theory**

| ADVANTAGES | DISADVANTAGES |
|---|---|
| • It makes planners and policy-makers think about their assumptions and challenge their beliefs about knowledge and learning.<br>• It can be applied in a variety of contexts.<br>• It provides a framework for categorising knowledge and agents.<br>• It can help to provide more detailed analysis of research evidence.<br>• It suggests new possibilities or options for change.<br>• It provides a more complete picture of forces affecting change. | • It neglects the ethical and emotional dimensions of leadership and management.<br>• It conflates description and prescription at the expense of analysis.<br>• It sometimes confuses explanation with prediction.<br>• It can be relativist.<br>• It advocates self-organisation and as such risks exonerating leaders and managers from accountability and responsibility. |

This theory is also relevant to building a community of learning for community health. Community health faculty leaders should understand the significance of the relationships and tensions in the midst of change to be able to build effective community of learning structures and programmes that improve learning in community. They must understand the political, analytical, and communication skills required to function effectively in these systems. As can be seen, this is consistent with the suggestions of the cultural analysis model, which Chapter 12 presents as a useful approach to identifying such professional development needs for community health education. Also, Chapter 13 on development of teaching and learning centres in community health, in particular, demonstrates the great importance community health educators/managers and communities tend to place on the fundamental characteristics of complex adaptive systems theory- autonomous agents, network structures, and profuse experimentation- in the process of developing teaching and learning centres in the community.

**Summary**

This chapter has presented the main suggestions or assumptions of several examples of leadership and management theories that provide understanding leading to effective building of a community of learning. There are several leadership and management theories that can be categorised into micro–level theories and macro-level theories. Micro-level theories help explain and predict individual behaviour (e.g. motivation theories) and interpersonal issues (e.g. leadership theories, communication theories, and theories of group dynamics). Macro-level theories explain issues at a broader, agency level. These theories focus on the best ways to organise work, on how to obtain the resources necessary to accomplish agency goals, on organisational level change, and on power dynamics. For the purpose of building a community of learning for community health, it is important for community health faculty leaders and consultants to also know which form of organisational structure will best promote the efficient achievement of organisational goals.

Thus, some important organisational-level theories that are particularly relevant for community health/PHC interventions and building a community of learning have also been covered, such as structural contingency theory, institutional theory, resource dependence theory and systems theories. These leadership and management theories are useful for community health faculty leaders to help them place their leadership functions in perspective. They should use them as frameworks on which to build their leadership styles which suit them, the environments in which they function, and the people they lead. In the following final chapter in Part One, we will look at how to build a community of learning for community health for the 21st century.

# 7

# *Building a Community of Learning Framework*

Despite community being so crucial for student learning in higher education, today learning in community has diminished due to several factors. These include expansion of large public institutions to accommodate government-mandated support of larger enrolments, leading to the emphasis of efficiency in structuring processes and to larger class sizes; increasing demands on faculty for research productivity outside the classroom and community learning environments, and increasing numbers of off-campus students Bickford et al (2010). The faculty leader and his/her team can rebuild the notion of community, thereby strengthening learning. Bickford et al (2010) describe three ways through which this can be done: (i) learning space design, (ii) information technology, community and information exchange and, (iii), pedagogical, curricular and co-curricular design for learning. The faculty leader and his or her team need to explore how building a community helps the creation of spaces for learning (and conversely, how creating learning-centred spaces can enhance their ability to build a community of learning); how technology can foster community and information exchange; and how community can foster learning through curricular, co-curricular and pedagogical design. This chapter deals with the building of a community of learning framework. It begins with descriptions of three strategic processes of building a community of learning. Then, it outlines six good practices in design processes of developmental interventions including the concepts of self reliance and sustainability as they relate to the building of the community of learning.

**Building a Community of Learning Framework**

The three strategic processes through which the community health education leader and his/her team can rebuild a community of learning are outlined by Bickford et al (2010) as follows:

**1. Learning Space Design**

- This is about designing new learning places that encourage communication rather than distance.
- It includes a community of facilities managers, faculty, student development professionals, administrators, architects, students, technologists and other stakeholders.
- It involves a process of discussion and innovation to create spaces that will re-engage students and staff in the teaching and learning process.
- This multiple view is required by the complex students' projects to give the needed information for making informed decisions in team learning.

Bickford et al offer five steps to harness the full potential of community and to engage community in co-creating the built learning environment:

**(1) Inviting stakeholders to contribute**

- Invite people with various views to participate in decision-making on learning space design.

**(2) Selecting and empowering a gifted leader**

- Select a leader who can build community as well as create settings safe for participation and team learning.
- He or she should have vision, empathy and should be able to listen and value various perspectives.
- He or she must be empowered to carry out the needed tasks.
- He or she should be able to empower others.

**(3) Understanding and respecting different views**

- This includes inviting students and faculty input on learning space design.
- It includes encouraging participation of individuals and understanding of differences in views, culture, power and hierarchy and urging sensitiveness to those dissimilarities.

**(4) Eradicating barriers to community learning**

- This includes preventing obstruction of collaboration in community learning by various communication styles and values of actors in the education process.
- It includes dealing with differences in knowledge and expertise, personality differences and group dynamics.
- It includes dealing with barriers that come from processes and systems that can prevent consensus formation (for example, determining who should fund the building of an integrated living-learning centre, academics or residential areas) (Bickford et al 2010).

**(5) Balancing performance and patience**

- This involves exercising patience to encourage new ideas to grow.
- However, endless discussion and debate should not be allowed as it can be

time-consuming and costly.
- Past accomplishments should be considered when designing new learning space models to avoid costly mistakes.

**2. Technology, Community, and Information Exchange**
- This involves delivering academic programmes or conducting face-to-face classes in various physical spaces using technology in or out of the space.
- In these learning situations technology should be used to foster learning through building community as well as creating and sharing knowledge within the group, while allowing interaction to take place in and outside the formal classroom setting.
- ICTs can foster community by making communication outside the classroom richer and more extensive, and classroom time free for more active learning approaches.
- Using ICTs students can research or write papers while networking to build community.
- Communication tools such as enterprise-level e-mail and calendaring as well as learning management systems are important tools for learning and information exchange.
- However, there is a surprising lag in the widespread development and adoption of applications that allow the spontaneous and ad-hoc teaming, which characterises an active community.
- The planning of physical space must consider the fact that face-to-face classroom meetings will become less didactic and more active, which encourages student participation and engagement in original learning approaches.

**3. Pedagogical, Curricular, and Co-curricular Design**
- This involves students engaging in many activities to form the social interactions needed to establish and build community.
- Students can achieve this without important faculty involvement, or faculty can shape, contribute to, and extend the learning environment of students.
- Professional development opportunities provide faculty the chance to experience student life again, which makes them value the possibilities of a learning community.
- Learning communities are increasingly common in faculty development programmes, where they provide a valuable learning process for those engaged in knowledge generation/production.
- Learning communities encourage open discussion and sharing among faculty and other stakeholders in the educational process.
- Learning communities assist participants deal with questions that relate to the nature of students and how they can be helped to learn.
- Learning and teaching centres in higher education provide strong mechanisms for stimulating institutional change that encompasses pedagogical, curricular, and co-curricular approaches which include faculty learning communities, experimental classrooms, support of student learning, and evaluation of stu-

dent learning.

- Teaching and learning centres advance partnerships between student development and faculty by, for instance, preparing faculty to facilitate learning in community, where they can serve as valuable change agents for the curricular, pedagogical and co-curricular innovations that advance community.

Thus, according to Bickford et al, building a community of learning can be achieved through three forms of strategic instruments that can advance learning through the community processes of designing spaces that support learning, using information and communication technologies, and designing structures for learning that include pedagogy, curricular and co-curricular programming. They are: (1) learning space design, which involves inviting people with various perspectives in participatory decision-making, selecting and empowering a talented leader who is able to tap into the potential of community, understanding and appreciating differences in perspective in decision-making, eliminating roadblocks to community learning, and balancing patience and performance; (2) technology, community, and information exchange, with particular reference to the role of communication in building a community of learning, and use of information and communication technologies in building a community of learning and; (3) pedagogical, curricular, and co-curricular design, focusing on faculty planned pedagogical, curricular, and co-curricular activities, students' creation of learning activities that foster a community of learning, professional development opportunities that strengthen a community of learning, and the role of learning and teaching centres in building a community of learning.

**Six Good Practices in Design Processes of Development Interventions**

Complementing and supporting the above plan are six good practices in any design process of a development intervention (IFAD 2011):

- Involving stakeholders who can usefully participate in the design.
- Conducting a comprehensive situational analysis with primary stakeholders to have a better knowledge of the context as a basis for designing the relevant building strategy and implementation and evaluation processes.
- Creating a logical and achievable building strategy that clearly indicates the goal and objectives that will be achieved together with the anticipated outputs and activities.
- Agreeing and focusing on cross-cutting issues such as poverty, gender and participation.
- Planning for long-term capacity development and sustainability to make sure that the project adds to the empowerment and self-reliance of local people and institutions.
- Building in opportunities and actions that enhance learning and make possible adaptation of the project strategy during implementation.

These actions are crucial in planning, implementing and evaluating the building process of a community of learning in the complex environment of community health where, as we have seen, the educational focus are the major health problems of a country where graduates of the programmes function. The implications of this are that: (1) the content of the programmes does not only rest on the discipline that contributes to them, but also on the problems that characterise the programmes (2) the specific nature of the main health problems in a particular population differentiates one programme from another (3) as problems change from time to time, so also programmes are highly oriented to changes in the environment and (4) the student activities in the programmes should include issues in health education and promotion, disease prevention, health research and involvement of people in improvement of their health status.

As discussed, such an education must be a process that is transformative and developmental. Within an environmental plan, such education can take place at the various levels of an individual, organisation, community and population. But in all instances the learning is conditional on engagement and is socially structured, and both formal and informal forms of learning are emphasised. As we have suggested, such education should rest on the Social Reconstructionism ideology which is grounded on the idea that education is a means of improving society. We have also indicated that in higher education communities, in which community members are committed to communicating with one another on an ever deeper and more authentic level, include communities of practice that involve groups of students, faculty and community members who work together, learn from each other and develop a common understanding of how to accomplish learning in a community. All these reflect the six good design practices of development interventions discussed earlier.

Many attempts to introduce educational interventions in community health have failed because such attempts have been made without due regard to such development practices. Why are these practices in building a community of learning for community health necessary? To begin with, many educational interventions in the community take some time to commence after initial design, during which the context will have changed. The development cycle usually includes many steps that lead to start-up, each of which takes time. Secondly, the initial design of the interventions may be attempted with limited time and resources. Many of the implementing partners will not have been identified and so there will have been limited participation in the process. This suggests a comprehensive participatory process of reviewing and, if need be, improving the design which is crucial at the beginning of the plan. After start-up, there are opportunities for improving the intervention design, such as on an annual basis as part of the annual progress review and planning process, and during the mid-term review. Chapters 8, 11 and 13 in Part Two describe community projects on learning space design, designing online cooperative and collaborative learning, and development of teaching and learning centres, respectively, that recognise the importance of such development cycles.

The concept of self-reliance which is included in the six good practices in designing a development intervention is important to consider as it is one of the bases of effective community health development in many countries, especially in sub-Saharan Africa. In fact, the concept of self-reliance is located centrally within the discourse of community development and is connected to related concepts like self-help, mutual-help, indigenous participation and rural development. Self-help, for example, enables the local people to exploit to their advantage resources, which would otherwise lie dormant and thereby perpetuate the ignorance and poverty of their community, by making use of the under-utilised labour. For instance, self-help for community development can increase the competence and confidence of a community in handling its affairs.

Developing skills for self-help is a prerequisite for survival in the modern world (Galtung et al 1980, cited by Fonchingong et al 2003). Self-help initiatives enable the people to rally local resources and efforts for development. This is especially appropriate to the concept of community development, which stresses the importance of people increasing their sense of responsibility, and taking assistance as just supplementary, but never replacing popular initiatives or local efforts (e.g. Fonchingong et al 2003)). The emphasis is on democratising with reliance on what people can do for themselves. The principle of self-help incorporates into the community development process the means of offering ordinary citizens the opportunity to share in making important decisions about their living conditions. This approach echoes the people-centredness of community development-attempts at satisfying felt needs (e.g, Fonchingong et al 2003). This entails community participation at all levels of intervention development.

The self-reliance concept advocates the need for people to improve their physical, social and other conditions using local initiatives and resources available. Self-reliance is quickly being accepted as a new formula for community development (e.g. Fonchingong et al 2003). Its widespread acceptance in development planning of most African countries has the tendency to give greater stimulus and cohesiveness to community development in these countries (e.g. Fonchingong et al 2003). Self-reliance is now seen as an important point of take-off for better living. The emphasis is to involve groups of people in planned programmes from which they may gain skills that will enable them to cope more successfully with the problems of their everyday life. Self-reliance is therefore considered to be development on the basis of a country's (region's) own resources, involving its population based on the potential of its cultural values and traditions. Individuals, groups and communities define their own development according to their own needs, values and aspirations.

Another concept that also has much relevance for building a community of learning for community health and is, as can be seen, featured in the six good practices of any developmental intervention is sustainability. There are different views about what sustainability means and what can be done to foster it. Sustainability is generally seen as an economic, social and ecological concept, which is a means of configuring civilisation and human activity (e.g. WCED 1987). It aims at providing for the best for humankind and the environment both now and in the future (e.g. WCED 1987).

The original term is sustainable development (UNCED 1992). Some experts now object to the term sustainable development as an umbrella term since it implies continued development that will cause great harm to humans in the future

(UNCED 1992). In contrast, sustainability integrates environmental, economic and social concerns. Sustainability, then, is nowadays applied as a criterion to evaluate all aspects of human activity (UNCED 1992). Ben Eli (2005/2006), for example, proposes a somewhat different concept of sustainability as an organising principle to enhance a well-functioning alignment between individuals, the economy, society and the regenerative capacity of the planet's life-supporting ecosystems. This alignment, according to Ben Eli, represents a specific kind of balance in the interaction between a population and the carrying capacity of its environment. Ben Eli suggests that it is this particular balance which must be the focus of a meaningful definition of sustainability. This concept of sustainability is based on five core principles that are expressed in relation to five fundamental domains shown in Box 12:

**Box 12: Sustainability: Five Fundamental Domains**

1. **The Material Domain:** Constitutes the basis for regulating the flow of materials and energy that underlie existence.
2. **The Economic Domain**: Provides a guiding framework for creating and managing wealth.
3. **The Domain of Life**: Provides the basis for appropriate behaviour in the biosphere.
4. **The Social Domain**: Provides the basis for social interactions.
5. **The Spiritual Domain**: Identifies the necessary attitudinal orientation and provides the basis for a universal code of ethics.

*Source: Ben Eli (2005/2006)*

In economics, sustainable growth consists of increases in real incomes (i.e. "inflation" -adjusted) or output that could be sustained for long periods of time (Department for the Environment, Food and Rural Affairs 2009). Therefore sustainable growth means, among other things, making profit. Social sustainability is concerned with the maintenance of social and human capital and keeping social and human capital intact. Human capital consists of knowledge, disposition, skills and expertise of people belonging to an organisation. It is a source of creativity and innovation, and therefore of the competitive advantage of an organisation (Woodcraft 2012).

In considering the concept of human capital increasing importance has now been given by theorists and analysts to the role of human learning within organisations and communities. Closely linked to the idea of learning or capital in organisations is the notion of social capital, which has gained importance among analysts in the current decade (OECD 2007)). Social capital refers to the components of social life, namely, the existence of networks, policies, institutions, relationships and norms (OECD 2007). A concept of social capital proposed by Putnam (1993) has three components, namely, moral obligations and norms, social values (particularly trust) and social networks (especially voluntary associations). The central tenet of this concept is that if a region successfully accumulates social capital it will have a well-functioning economic system and a high level of political integration. Another idea of social capital postulated by Bourdieu (1986) emphasises conflicts and the power function- social relations that increase the ability of an actor to advance her/his interests. Also, Coleman (1988) explains the concept of social capital by identifying three forms of social capital: obligations and expectations which rest on the trustworthiness of the social environments, norms accompanied by sanctions, and information- flow capability of the social structure. According to Coleman (1988), the public good (a commodity or service that is provided without profit to all members of a society, either by the government or a private individual or organisation) component of social capital is a characteristic shared by most forms of social capital.

These aspects of social life enable people to act together, create synergies and build partnerships. There is a link between human and social capital. Social capital can influence the ability to acquire human capital through, for example, the enhancement of learning at school by strong communities (OECD 2007).

Also, in order to preserve social capital for sustained economic growth and development it is necessary to foster networks of trust and knowledge creation and sharing at the organisational, community and regional levels, as well as between different sectors, such as government, higher education and business (OECD 2005). Goodland et al (1996) argue that social capital requires the maintenance and replenishment of shared values by communities, social and religious groups.

Within the wider health sector, sustainability has become synonymous with self-sufficiency in financing and often applied to situations where external aid agencies sought to induce developing country governments to take on the responsibility for funding activities that previously had been donor funded (Levine et al 2001). However it is now generally agreed that both domestic and external funding are necesary for sustaining public health programme. Thus, the concepts of self-reliance and sustainability and the other ideas in the building of a community of learning frameworks are consistent with the democratic principles of participation, cooperation, empowerment, capacity building, etc., which define the concepts of community health and PHC and provide conceptual understanding of building a community of learning.

As will be seen, the concepts of self-reliance and sustainability are vital to the idea of building a community of learning in community health and are recurrent themes in the following chapters of the book.

**Summary**

This final chapter in part one has outlined the building of a community of learning framework that incorporates the theories, concepts, principles and conditions we had considered in previous chapters. It has also described a complementary scheme of good practices of designing any development intervention. In doing so, the chapter has considered the related concepts of self-reliance and sustainability as they are so important for the concept of community health and PHC and the building of a community of learning in this health environment. We have seen in this chapter that community health education leaders can build a community of learning for community health through three forms of strategic tools (Bickford et al 2010) that can advance learning through the community processes of designing spaces that support learning, using information technology, and designing structures for learning that include pedagogy, curricular and co-curricular programming. How the faculty leader handles these four strategic tools and what this means for the systems and structures of education and community health/PHC will be discussed in more detail in Part Two.

# PART TWO

## *Application of the concepts, theories and principles*

# 8

## *Learning space design*

Design generally refers to an organisational arrangement, or structure of elements, parts, or details. In Part One, Chapter 7, we outlined a building of community of learning framework which includes learning space design. Six good practices in any design process of a development intervention were also outlined to support and complement the community of learning framework. Several education and learning theories, as well as leadership and management theories that are particularly relevant for community health interventions and designing learning spaces in the community were covered. Part One also looked at theories, concepts and principles that are related to technology, community and information exchange to enhance a community of learning. We will now discuss how community health educators and their partners can be involved in designing learning spaces in community health to ensure that these and the other conditions we have described are present in the learning space design process.

This chapter outlines several perspectives for achieving this, highlighting how these perspectives can be used in designing learning spaces in community health drawing from the concepts outlined in Part One and giving examples from general education, community-oriented health professional education and management and leadership fields. The chapter starts with the issue of involving stakeholders in learning space design. It then looks at how to analyse the current context for learning spaces with particular reference to community health education. It describes the roles of education, educational technology, information services, and facilities management and planning in the design of learning spaces in the community. It outlines the steps in the learning space project design. Finally, the chapter discusses suggestions and approaches that are useful for designing learning environments that can foster a community of learning for community health.

**Stakeholders**

As indicated in Part One, Chapter 7, learning space design involves inviting people with various perspectives in participatory decision-making, selecting and empowering a talented leader who is able to tap into the potential of community, understanding and appreciating differences in perspectives in decision-making, eliminating barriers to community learning, and balancing patience and performance.

Designing a good health development intervention like designing learning spaces as a component of building a community of learning for the education of health professionals in the community requires careful attention to the social processes and institutional development that will enable learning and the empowerment of primary stakeholders. Community health educators and their partners implementing such interventions without good stakeholder consultation are setting themselves up for failure. Those who do consult widely increase their chances of success.

Stakeholder is a person who has something to gain or lose through the outcomes of a planning process, programme or project (Friedman et al 2006). There are several reasons why involving stakeholders in learning space design is important specifically for: (1) inspiring them to identify, manage and control their own development aspirations, and so empower themselves (2) ensuring the goals and objectives of the design will be relevant and, as a result, meet the real needs of the community (3) ensuring the project strategy is appropriate to local circumstances (4) building the partnerships and ownership (5) although time-consuming in the development stage, inviting people with various perspectives in participatory decision-making is at the end less time-consuming than leaving them out, and (6) local participation early on can also be cost-effective in the long run.

Thus it is necessary, as a first step in learning space design, to carry out an initial stakeholder analysis. Stakeholder Analysis is a technique used to identify and assess the influence and importance of key people, groups of people, or organisations that may significantly impact the success of your activity or project (Friedman et al 2006).This requires listing potential stakeholders, prioritising who must be involved and deciding with them the nature of their involvement. Such stakeholders are the individuals, groups or institutions that are involved in or are concerned about student learning in the community. This exercise is the foundation for understanding stakeholder needs. As public participation becomes increasingly embedded in national and international public health policy (Hughes et al 2008), it becomes ever more crucial for decision-makers to understand who is affected by these decisions and the actions they take, and who has the power to influence their outcome: the stakeholders.

A technique to help identify which individuals or organisations to include in the learning space design project is known as a 'stakeholder analysis' (Friedman et al 2006). The following stages have been identified to support the stakeholder analysis process:

- Identify and map internal and external stakeholders
- Assess the nature of each stakeholder's influence and importance

- Construct a matrix to identify stakeholder influence and importance
- Monitor and manage stakeholder relationships

Stakeholder participation in teaching and learning space design in the community should involve working with local communities or valuing their views above others. It also entails understanding differences within and between local communities, which means that community health educators should listen keenly and work together to gain insights into local relationships and interests. With some creativity it is possible to include the poorest, most isolated and illiterate of groups. An important purpose of teaching and learning centres in community health, which Chapter 13 deals with, can be to strengthen community health-related municipal administration and civil society organisations in non-literate and geographically isolated communities. Such a community participatory process can create the opportunity for primary stakeholders to adjust part of a teaching and learning centre project design strategy to make them suitable to their situation and therefore more likely to meet their real needs. As discussed in Part One, Chapter 2, Freire's (2000) description of the oppressed resonates so well with how the role of community members are often seen by health educators and officials concerning community health projects and programmes. For example, we have seen that despite the majority of health science schools developing community-oriented experiences for learners to prepare them for their role in community health practice, these experiences situated away from universities do not sufficiently involve the community in their planning (Unverzagt et al 1998). Freire advises encouraging participation of individuals and groups in such community health education projects and programmes.

As discussed in Chapter 7, for a community health education leader engaged in learning space design to be able to tap into the potential of community, he or she must possess certain qualities. The leadership and management theories we outlined in Part One, Chapter 6, are important in identifying the qualities of the leader as they help us to understand the conditions that make a leader in community health education realise his or her potential. As we have seen in the chapter, Orlando's model of nursing focuses on the need for one to function as a leader and partner by working with community members to identify community health needs and needed policies and programmes. The model also suggests that the client should be included in every step of decision making about care, thereby making the process of care becoming more of a partnership. What is also required here is a transformational leader who motivates followers to achieve a vision that matches their values. The leader influences others to work towards achieving something new, like a new dream that has not yet been imagined. He/she is capable of changing the situation to one that is unlike the status quo. Such leaders are needed in teaching and learning agencies to create cultures that support ongoing learning, experimentation, and creation of new knowledge, as well as promote a culture of safety and positive work and learning environments for others (Orlando 1990; Burns 1978).

To select such a leader who is influenced by these conditions, techniques like the Analytic Hierarchy Process (AHP) (Saaty 2012) structured technique for organising and analysing such a complex decision can be used. It has particular application in group decision making and is used around the world in a wide variety of decision-making situations, in fields such as government, business, industry, health care, and education.

As previously discussed in Chapter 7, a number of barriers limits communication in higher education (such as different communication styles and values), which a faculty leader should deal with. This is also the case in health care where there are well-developed politics described by Boaden et al (1999): (i) one aspect is professional representation to governments and other agencies to advance their interests. Professionals have been successful in this endeavour, but the political processes involved are becoming harder, hence there is a need to change the ability or skills of the professional health worker. (ii) The other aspect is the area of public/community health where specialist doctors do not treat patients and have comparatively little to do with many of the health workers who provide direct health care to communities. Their principal role lies in modifying public and institutional behaviour in ways that agree with prevention of disease and promotion of health. They have been doing this work for a long time; however, the influence they command require high understanding and skills in policy and decision – making processes, and processes of institutional operations. Furthermore, the type of reward which comes from the cure and alleviation of patients' conditions and their patients' appreciation is reduced in the PHC system, because the link between health professionals' efforts and the health of the people is less clear (Boaden et al 1999). There is often a hierarchical order in health systems that rest on prestige and power between the different medical traditions. This situation often results in more powerful traditions (e.g. medical doctors) exploiting or suppressing feeble traditions (e.g. traditional healers).

We also saw in Chapter 7 that differences in knowledge and expertise, personality and group dynamics, can also present roadblocks to a community of learning. The team leader and teachers need to influence decisions that can bring about changes in structural arrangements, expenditure patterns, organisational, and administrative structures that are needed for designing learning space effectively. The processes of consultation in such efforts are often quite unusual for the majority of health professionals and the close association between those involved can bring about traditional behaviour linked to hierarchy. Therefore, establishing trust, respect and egalitarian partnership can be a long and difficult process. The faculty leader trying to encourage communities to participate in designing learning space may have to deal with many constraints, such as professional monopolisation of health services leading to loss in community participation and learning in community. Learning to tackle such difficulties will help the leader and teachers increase and strengthen their teaching capacity, as well as serve as role models to their students. Therefore, it is important for the leader and his/her team to take a comprehensive situational analysis of the current context for learning spaces in the community.

## Situational Analysis of Current Context for Learning Spaces in Community Health Education

**The situation analysis involves:**

- Learning as much as possible about the project context and the interests and needs of local people.
- Using tools, such as a problem tree that is good for simple situations, or a problem-based planning which conforms well with a more mechanical approach to solving problems instead of facilitating local development processes.
- Analysing future visions to indicate opportunities for improvement and achievements that can be further enhanced.

Community health educators should use an approach or approaches that suit their particular situations. To be useful or effective, a situation analysis should:

- Bring together information gathering and analysis concerning the local environment, participatory processes like participatory appraisals, multi-stakeholder workshops, community meetings and expert advice.
- Provide more insights about the stakeholder situation and have better capacity to design a solid learning space project. However, this will not be achieved in one community meeting. People's perspectives evolve as they debate and listen.
- Provide continuous dialogue, after a community meeting that can lead to improvements in project design. Therefore, the leader should ensure that the situation analysis is designed as a series of events.

Community health educators and their partners may wish to carry out a situation analysis exercise by brainstorming ideas and concepts round learning spaces that occur under the following headings (American Association of Medical Colleges (AAMC 2008):

**Educational Trends**

- Flexibility
- Team-based learning
- Learning communities
- Display technologies
- Interactivity
- Distance learning
- Computer-based testing
- Lecture cast (audio-video)
- Facilities fee

**Economic Climate**

- Budget cuts
- Student debt
- Business model

- Facilities fee

**Political Factors**
- Public expectation
- Space ownership/competition
- Programme ownership
- Practice culture
- Students in community

**Technology Factors**
- Rapidly changing technology
- Structural capacity for technology
- New interfaces
- High definition/standards(+-)

**Customer Needs**
- 24/7 Access
- Internet access
- Accreditation/certification
- Staffing
- Faculty development/user training
- Teaching styles
- Learning styles
- Study preference

**Uncertainties or Unknowns**
- Budgets
- Curricular change
- Class size (+-)
- Rapidly changing technology

The following are key themes, questions and methods (International Fund for Agricultural Development (Infad) 2011) that the design leader and his/her team can adopt for a detailed situation analysis with stakeholders:

**Key themes, questions and methods (italicised) for a detailed situation analysis with stakeholders**

**Stakeholders** *(stakeholder maps, institutional diagrams, secondary data)*
- Who are the local people likely to benefit from the project?
- Who are the other key stakeholders?
- How do different stakeholder groups interact?
- What are the power relations between different groups?

**Problems and Issues** *(rich pictures, conceptual maps, focus group discussions, historical analyses, secondary data, matrix ranking)*

- What problems or issues are central to the focus of the project?
- What are the main problems or concerns of the different stakeholder groups and how do these relate to the focus of the project?

**Visions and Opportunities** *(rich pictures, role plays)*
- What changes would different stakeholder groups like to see the project bring about?
- Generally, what visions, hopes or dreams do different stakeholders have and are there implications for the project?
- What opportunities do stakeholders see for realising their visions?

**Biophysical Setting** *(maps, transects, field visits, seasonal calendars)*
- What are geographical characteristics of the project areas?
- What are the climatic conditions?
- What are the main forms of land use?
- What are the environmental problems or risks?

**Organisations** *(institutional diagrams, network diagrams, flow charts, matrix ranking)*
- What are the important government, business and NGO organisations?
- How effectively are these organisations performing?
- How are the different organisations linked together? (Power relations, communications, joint work, competitors)

**Infrastructure** *(resource maps)*
- What are the key infrastructure issues for the area?

**Legal, Policy and Political Institutions** *(rich pictures, institutional diagrams, historical analyses, focus group interviews, secondary data)*
- What legal factors are significant for the project?
- What government policies and programmes are significant?
- What are the main government and political structures and processes in the area?

**Economic** *(well-being ranking, daily activity charts, seasonal calendars, secondary data)*
- What is the economic situation of local people?
- What are the main forms of economic livelihood?
- What at are the key characteristics of the local economy?
- What are the market opportunities and constraints?

**Social & Cultural** *(historical analysis, focus group discussions, SWOT analysis)*
- What are the main social and cultural conditions relevant to the project?

*Source: IFAD (2011)*

As already mentioned, one reason why it is particularly crucial to involve stakeholders in teaching and learning centre design is to ensure that the design strategy is appropriate to local circumstances. With a good understanding of the situation, the leader and his/her team are now ready to start developing the project design strategy. This simply explains clearly what everyone hopes to achieve and how it will be achieved. A project strategy includes the objective hierarchy, implementation arrangements and resources required. These important elements of the project design are considered in the final sections of this chapter dealing with the steps and phases of the project design. However, in order to successfully design physical spaces that serve current and future learning and assessment needs it is necessary to use the expertise of a broad range of individuals, many of whom may not have known each other before the project. Each expert brings a specific perspective and vision for the space and its purpose. The following section presents a description of the roles of key stakeholders in the learning space design team and process (AAMC 2008) with information from the relevant literature.

## The Roles of Education, Educational Technology, Information Services, and Facilities Management and Planning in the Design of learning Spaces for Community Health Education

### The Role of Education

The role of education is to ensure that decisions are made that result in a physical environment joined with current and future needs for learning and/or assessment such as education trends (e.g. flexibility, interactivity, learning strategies like team-based learning, cooperative/collaborative learning and telemedicine ) The clinics and health centres in which doctors, nurses, midwives, students, etc, collaborate can be better redesigned to be responsive to the learning elements of the situation analysis. For instance, space flexibility allows the clinics and health centres to concurrently accommodate different users. Usually, these spaces might simultaneously support student learning in various aspects of primary health care and community health including appropriate technology, traditional medicine, etc. Boaden et al (1999), for example, describe a useful model of four educational stages for learning clinical skills in the community that demonstrates the support to learning that can be included in the planning of student learning in the community through redesigned community facilities (These steps are described in some detail in Chapter 10). Community health educators need to be actively involved in the decision-making process to prevent decisions being made based on cost, feasibility, and style without due regard to the community health learning facility's chief educational aims.

In short, educators need to be actively involved in the decision-making process of the design. They should concentrate on learning outcomes, providing internal summaries, asking for clarification throughout the process, and assessing the abilities of the space to ensure that space design decisions pay particular attention to learning outcomes.

**The Role of Educational Technology**

There are significant advances in community health and the education of health professionals for the community that demand the creation and support of more diverse and complex technology in learning spaces in the community than ever before. The education of health professionals for community health is increasingly moving beyond planning for instruction in on-campus facilities and resources to greater use of new learning space with ICTs for learning (e.g. Intel World Ahead Programme 2010). As we mentioned in Part One, Chapter 1, for instance, studies in community health are focusing on how the built environment and socio-economic status affect health. ICT applications like video/teleconfer-

Figure 4: Elements of a Sustainable Project

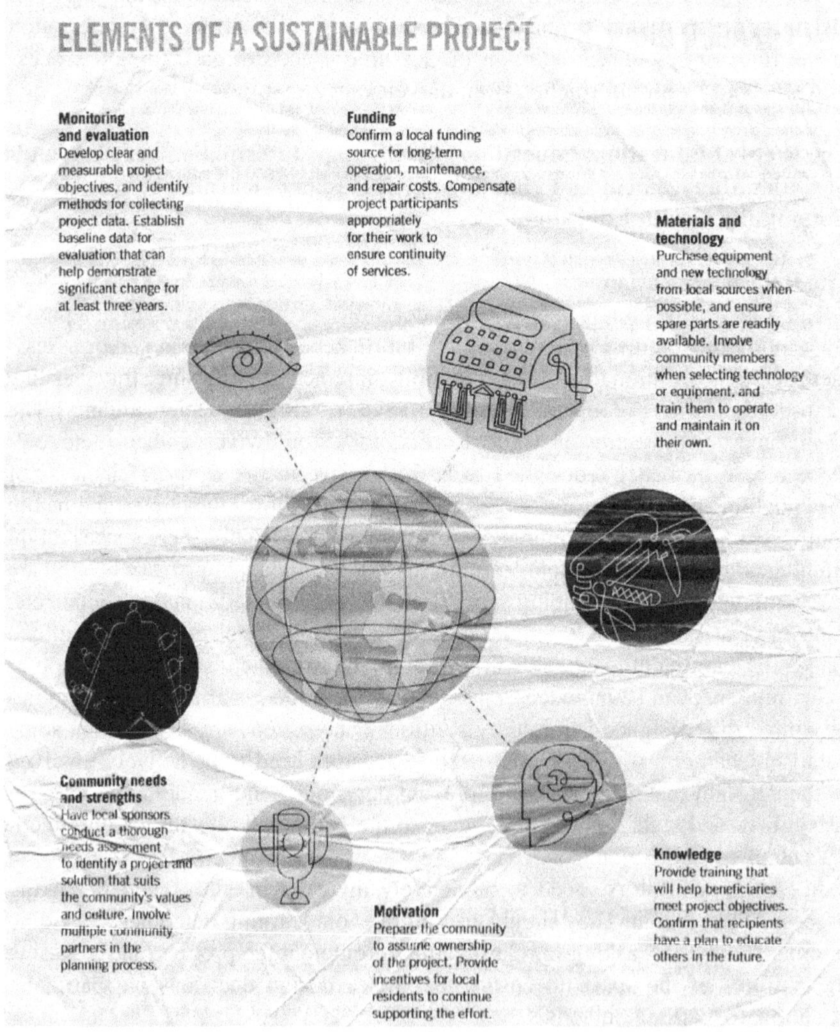


*Source: Rotary International (2012)*

encing, telemedicine (which as already mentioned is proving to be so useful in community health education) and the new District Health Information System (DHIS) tool which has now been adopted in many PHC Systems are technologies that can now be usefully included in learning space design in community health. The significance of all this is that the educational technologists now play a critical role in the planning of any learning space, and this role is becoming bigger and more complex.

The educational technologist's role in the learning space design process is important for several reasons:

- His/her understanding of how technology is used in a particular space and can advice on the selection, placement and use of technology.
- His/her background and training enables him to speak strongly and consistently on behalf of students and teachers in terms of their educational needs.
- He/she gives daily support to faculty and students to integrate technology into their teaching.
- He/she ensures that learning space is designed appropriately and that the technology supports the teaching and learning process.

He/she does these by:

a) Conducting observational visits and interviews in present learning spaces to see how technology is being used, misused, or not used at all.

b) Providing photos that can give architects, furniture designers, and other members of the design team significant information that can help in designing better learning spaces.

c) Documenting several scenarios of what happens in the space in a day, considering the various activities and times of year, to get an insight into key design issues that go beyond a specific teaching session.

d) Piloting new technologies. Vendors may be willing to loan and install equipment from their seed pools, as well as provide training and support

This account demonstrates an example (Web 2012: 1) of such partnership:

MidCity Office Furniture recently completed the space planning, design, and furniture installation for Community Health Centre of Buffalo's new facility at 34 Benwood Avenue in Buffalo. The facility represents a $6 million investment in the community. MidCity used Colecraft, Global, First Office, OFS, and Offices to Go tables and seating as well as First Office lounge seating to create a space that was comfortable and inviting to the community, while still maintaining the functionality and technology of a high-quality medical care facility. "Community Health has already noticed that the space's flexibility and functionality are allowing them to better meet the needs of their patients and community," says Kurt Amico, President of MidCity Office Furniture.

Collaboration in various forms in the execution of curriculum policy such as borrowing staff, sharing ideas, and favouring exchange does pay dividends. It is needless to waste time developing a product if someone else can do it better for you or with you. Different types of organisations are good at different kinds of things, which give a place a better chance of survival. Therefore, the educational technologist should visit other institutions that have similar types of spaces to gather information that will be helpful in making decisions about learning space elements, such as communication devices.

We saw in Part One, Chapter 7 that support and sustainability are featured in the six good practices of any developmental intervention. As we noted there, the concepts of self-reliance and sustainability and the other ideas in the building of community of learning frameworks are consistent with the democratic principles of participation, cooperation, empowerment, capacity building, etc., which define the concepts of community health and PHC and provide a conceptual understanding of the building of a community of learning process. It is therefore crucial to have both support and sustainability models agreed to before any final decisions are made on technology purchasing, guided by these principles, for example, budget for regular replacement of equipment. The idea must be to include the levels of sustainability in the project design - economic, social, environmental, cultural and ethical. Figure 4 presents elements of a sustainable project that community health educators and their collaborators can usefully incorporate in their project designs.

**The Role of Information Services**

As we saw in Part One, Chapter 5, cognitive collaboration, for example, becomes operational when two or more people work interactively to develop a joint solution to a problem. Therefore, for all components to work well together, it is imperative that colleagues/ partners involved in information services be included in the design process early. This will facilitate integration of the appropriate technology infrastructure to ensure a successful outcome of the learning space design.

The role of information services includes making judgements about ICT infrastructure, data management, support services, and adaptability.

**(a) ICT Infrastructure**

This includes telephony network architecture, video, computer hardware, and integration with the mechanical plant. Points that must be kept in mind include:

- Using space that has its own data centre or using smaller machine rooms.
- Using standard server technology or a high-performance computing environment with chilled water feeds and increased electrical and HVAC capacity.
- Using a voice network standard support IP phones or a separate telephone infrastructure.
- Determining the impact of the general architectural design of the space on the location of wiring closets.
- The right balance of wired and wireless access points.
- The type of Uninterruptible Power Supply (UPS) required, the number of UPS, and whether used only for the education technology equipment or shared to support other equipment.

**(b) Data Management**

This includes decisions on where and how data generated within the learning space will be captured and stored. Here, points that must be thought about include:

- The creation of new data storage requirements by the use of computer-based tools in the learning space in the community. This may include connectivity to other school or university-based systems and access to systems inside and outside the community such as clinical partners, teaching and learning centres, and commodity internets.
- Other systems that will interact with the technology in the new space, such as exchanging data with existing Learning Management Systems, for example, Blackboard systems.
- The level of security that will be needed for spaces where data is stored. Here, consideration of the related national acts and requirements is crucial.

**( c ) Support Services**

This includes judgment on who provides the needed supports on technology. These are some indications of this:

- The day and time technology support comes from the school or university IT staff and if there are any conditions on the support, such as the choice of only one type of equipment.
- Persons expected to support the specific educational technology deployed in the space and what are the staffing requirements, for instance, the level of support the vendor will provide and for how long.
- Space required for operational controls of activities such as observation of clinical skills, and the technology needed.

**(d) Adaptability**

This includes thinking about how to make buildings adaptable to meet changing technology needs. Technology questions to be considered here include using the information services expertise of the architects and facilities professionals at the the beginning of the discussions to enhance flexible design. This approach also provides design teams the chance to know the kind of technology changes the information services team is planning in the near term.

Often the community health schools do not own the hospitals, clinics, health centres, teaching and learning centres and other community settings where faculty and students teach, learn, research and practise community health care. Thus, the schools rely on clinical partners to help deliver the right technology for the learning experience that is directly connected to patient care. Therefore, there is also need for cooperation and collaboration across all partners in these settings as already highlighted. This can be achieved through bi-monthly meetings that include representatives from community health schools, information services staff, the schools' facilities departments, etc. Such a standing committee or group meeting is designed to discuss all projects and ensure that there are open lines of communication. This, which can be additional to project team meetings, can help build a collaborative environment that encourages design team members work harmonously on projects. As already mentioned in Part One, Chapter 5, it is a good idea to have all stakeholders involved in learning space development projects as early as possible.

## The Role of Facilities Management and Planning

Community health schools may have planning and design professionals (architects, engineers, facility managers, etc.) on staff. Alternatively, they may have access to such professionals from their parent or collaborating institutions. These professionals have not only the background, but also the experience and responsibility to assist in the development of learning spaces. There are many reasons why they should be involved in the design process early:

- they have the experience and expertise to inform planning requirements
- they can serve as the overall guide of the project
- they can act as the steward for the facility in the future
- facility planners and managers can often identify space, land or funding for the project

A major consideration of the facilities manager and other planning team members is designing spaces that can facilitate cooperative/collaborative learning. Current teaching is mostly carried out in large mixed group settings like the lecture theatre. While such a setting has the economic benefits of size, it is disadvantageous for learning because of its anonymity and homogeneity of identity. It has been widely shown that this approach to learning is not only unproductive, it often leads to group of students ignoring one another and feelings of resentment that learning chances are being diluted. Rather than working in such large settings, students now prefer to work in pairs or small groups to carry out problem-solving tasks cooperatively (e.g. Szasz 1969)

Thus, in order to successfully design physical spaces that serve current and future learning and assessment needs, it is necessary to use the expertise of a broad range of individuals, many of whom may not have known one another before the project. Each expert brings a specific perspective and vision for the space and its purpose. For instance, the setting up of a telemedicine unit, which is increasingly proving to be an important communication tool in community health education, requires infrastructure such as an air-conditioned, sound-proof room with electrical outlets for connecting various equipment and a very good earthling pit.

The WHO defines Telemedicine as "The delivery of health care services, where distance is a critical factor, by all healthcare professionals using information and communication technologies for the exchange of valid information for diagnosis, treatment and prevention of disease and injuries, research and evaluation, and for the continuing education of healthcare providers, all in the interests of advancing the health of individuals and their communities," (WHO 2010: 8).

A facilities manager has a major responsibility for informing decisions on such infrastructure and equipment. There is need for video conferencing hardware (e. g. television), ICTs hardware (e.g. computer and printer) and connectivity hardware (e.g. satellite-based, such as VSATs (Very Small Aperture Terminals) for the unit. Perspectives on these are brought to the discussion by the ICT specialist. Also, there are various instrumentations that can be connected to the video-conferencing unit to directly relay data from the patient, such as Digital 12 lead ECG, Electronic stethoscope, Digital Microscope, Digital Blood Pressure Monitor, Skin camera, Doppler Ultrasound and Echocardiography equipment etc, on which a medical technologist should be able to give useful advice (e.g. American

Telemedicine Association (ATA) 2006)

The need to identify all stakeholders, to develop an overall project structure and approach, to build a consensus and understanding by all involved, and to raise expectations that are realistic in the process of developing learning spaces as early as possible cannot be overemphasised. It is important to obtain support and agreement early enough from the top echelons leaders of the organisation, together with identification of possible funding sources and supporters. The outcome of this early project stage is crucial as it will ultimately determine whether a project keeps to its schedule and budget, and is implemented as expected. Table 34, which educators seeking to build learning space in community health may find useful, demonstrates this and other normal steps in a learning space capital project design.

## Steps in the Learning Space Project Design

Project *need identification* is a repeatable process for documenting, validating, ranking and approving candidate projects within an organisation. Due to the changing financial conditions within the total organisation, it is necessary to establish a stable process for approving projects for initiation.

*Programming* is the way in which a project is planned. This involves listing all the operations that need to take place for the completion of construction and assigning them time duration. This then gives an overall programme for the work and the overall time it will take to complete the project.

In the *pre-design phase*, architects obtain necessary permits, determine estimated construction costs and develop construction timelines.

Architects refer to another phase of a building programme as the *schematic design phase*

(American Institute of Architects (AIA) 2007). It comes after the pre-design phase, during which an architect and an owner develop a written description of a construction project.

These four steps are the most crucial and each must be carried out as completely as possible and should mirror the agreement of the key stakeholders prior to going on to the next step. This must happen even if it means going back and re-doing aspects or the entire prior step. During these four steps the total project budget is developed and priorities are established on what needs to be included.

*Design development* is a transitional phase of an architect/engineer (A/E) services in which the design moves from the schematic design phase to the contract document phase. In this phase, the A/E prepares drawings and other presentation documents to crystallise the design concept and describe it in terms of architectural, electrical, mechanical, and structural systems. In addition, the A/E also prepares a statement of the probable project cost.

This activity can only commence after the Schematic Design and Cost Plan have been approved by the Department. Design development should resolve all outstanding design issues and address matters such as utility company negotiations, metering, monitoring and control systems, landscaping, water and waste management and way finding signage. A further capital cost estimate and recurrent operating costs will be prepared to demonstrate that the project is still within capital budget and recurrent estimates. If not, then alternative recommendations required to achieve the budget will have to be assessed and initiated.

A *design development report* will be prepared to demonstrate the issues of planning, design, materials selection, construction and constructability, staging, services integration and co-ordination, structural, civil, mechanical, electrical, hydraulic and energy services that should have been addressed and integrated into the proposal to ensure an effective project outcome. Typical documentation required at the completion of this stage is set out in a checklist and should include components such as the site plan, coordinated reflected ceiling plans, mechanical services including air conditioning, lifts, heating, ventilation, medical gases and plant rooms together with reticulation systems, equipment briefing schedules, energy, water and waste management systems including recycling facilities, recurrent cost estimates for operations and management, energy and resources and specifications, and supporting documents used during the completion of a construction project (e.g. Iowa State University 2013).

**Table 34: Typical capital project process for new construction and major renovations.**

| | | | | Central Campus Service Providers | | | | External Service Providers | | | | | |
|---|---|---|---|---|---|---|---|---|---|---|---|---|---|
| PROJECT PROCESS STEP | STAKEHOLDERS | Occupant / End User | Medical School Facilities Management and Planning Group | Planning and Project Management Group | Plant Maintenance and Operations Group | Other Service Providers eg. Public Safety, Environmental Health, Purchasing, etc. | Legal Counsel | Architectural and Engineering Consultants | Construction Management Consultants | Vendors | Contractors | Comments | Project Process Step Duration (months) |
| Need Identification | | 3 | 3 | 1 | 0 | 0 | 0 | 0 | 0 | 0 | 0 | End users working w/ their leadership w/assistance from Fac. Mgmt. staff | 6 to 12 |
| Programming | | 3 | 3 | 3 | 0 | 0 | 0 | 3 | 0 | 1 | 0 | | 1 to 6 |
| Pre Design / Concept Design | | 3 | 3 | 3 | 1 | 1 | 0 | 3 | 0 | 1 | 0 | | 3 to 9 |
| Schematic Design (SD) | | 3 | 3 | 3 | 1 | 1 | 0 | 3 | 0 | 1 | 0 | | 1 to 3 |
| Design Development (DD) | | 2 | 3 | 3 | 1 | 1 | 0 | 3 | 0 | 2 | 0 | | 3 to 6 |
| Construction Documentation (CD) | | 1 | 2 | 2 | 1 | 1 | 1 | 3 | 1 | 2 | 0 | | 6 to 12 |
| Bidding / Award of Contracts | | 1 | 2 | 3 | 0 | 1 | 1 | 2 | 1 | 1 | 2 | | 1 to 3 |
| Construction | | 1 | 1 | 2 | 1 | 1 | 0 | 2 | 3 | 2 | 3 | | 9 to 24 |
| Commissioning | | 1 | 2 | 2 | 2 | 2 | 0 | 3 | 2 | 1 | 2 | Should start during design and proceed through activation | 3 to 6 |
| Activation / Move-In | | 3 | 3 | 1 | 1 | 1 | 0 | 1 | 1 | 1 | 1 | | 1 to 3 |

Level of involvement: High = 3 Low = 1

Notes:
Major issues that impact duration of project process steps, overall project schedule duration, and level of stakeholder involvement
Project type, size, timing will determine project process step durations
Decision making and approval processes will determine overall duration of project

*Source: AAMC 2008*

Thus, designing a good health development intervention like designing learning spaces as a component of building a community of learning for the education of health personnel in the community requires careful attention to the social processes and institutional development that will enable learning and the empowerment of primary stakeholders. It demands a situation analysis that involves learning as much as possible about the project context and the interests and needs of local people in order to design a relevant project. This learning is best if done with several groups of stakeholders such as community health educators, educational technologists, information technologists and facilities managers (e.g. AAMC 2008). With a good understanding of the situation, the leader and his/her team are now ready to start developing the project design strategy. This, as we have seen, consists of the systematic steps of need identification, programming, pre-design/concept design,schematic designs (SD), design development (DD), and construction documentation (CD).

All these deal with the process of designing learning space with particular reference to building a community of learning in community health/PHC education. This, as we have seen, is an important component of the framework for building a community of learning. There is, however, the need to look further at the kind of learning space that should be produced by such a process - learning space that will meet the needs of community health and PHC. Part Two, Chapter 13 discusses this and other issues particularly in relation to the development of teaching and learning centres in the community. In the following and final section, we consider the types of learning environment designs that community health educators and other stakeholders can produce to foster a community of learning for community health.

**Considerations in Designing Learning Environments that Foster a Community of Learning for Community Health**

As already indicated, Bickford et al (2010), for instance, outline several examples of pedagogical and curriculum approaches to fostering community of learning. Table 35 demonstrates these approaches which include elements of cooperative/collaborative learning and the asynchronous and synchronous learning modes that are related to them. For example, the pedagogical approaches incorporate not only faculty learning about each other and from each other, but also projects involving students working in teams resulting in student presentation of projects, and class activities are improved by finishing a significant part of course requirements online. Also, for instance, curriculum activities include preparing students through online collaborative activities using websites, mentoring students, students' research projects that lead to presentations and service- learning projects.

But most crucially, the table presents several suggestions on how to design the learning environment to foster community of learning, based on the examples of pedagogical and curriculum approaches. These include removing the lectern to create open spaces and interaction between students and between students and lecturers, arranging the seats in the environment to allow for easy movement of students and teachers, using learning management systems that give delivery of course material online thereby facilitating exchange of messages, etc, and facilitation of student and faculty interaction by web-based resources that make face-to-face meetings more important. They also include establishment of learning support centres for providing additional tutoring that are spacious and equipped with gadgets such as computers, research laboratories, libraries and faculty workspaces used as learning spaces that promote brainstorming meetings, and physical environments that enhance interaction between visitors on campus and those off campus.

Table 35 presents pedagogical and curriculum approaches, as well as the suggested corresponding learning environment designs that are similar to teaching and learning methods which, according to Boaden et al (1999), are used for learning in the community. Boaden et al (1999) classify such methods into two categories. One category includes all the methods and techniques suited to teaching and learning activities in the classroom and covers class discussion, small group work and the lecture. These can range from educational activities in a formal setting to highly interactive self-study or group learning employing open learning materials or computers. The other category includes methods that mainly aim to use experience as the basis for learning and encompasses clinical activities, as well as activities based on fieldwork within the wider community. As we will see later, methods in the two categories, particularly methods such as group learning can be so useful in building a community of learning in community health. But as the discussion shows, the proposed approaches, together with the plans to change the learning environment require a change in health care and education systems including attitudes and the manner we plan and manage such educational innovations in the community if they are to meet the requirements of a community health-centric education.

Clearly, many of the approaches proposed in Table 35 may require considerable investment in development. Development costs are related to issues like constructing buildings, purchasing hardware and software, as well as developing programmes and transferring programmes to new media (e.g. CD-ROM) in especially health centres and clinics where community health education are often delivered). Many developing countries may not be able to meet these requirements because of their resource-constrained environments. As we have seen in Part One , Chapter 2, and in chapters of Part Two, one factor that is reducing the gains registered by PHC in such countries is the influence of microeconomic forces resulting in weakening of healthcare systems due to fiscal austerity and the loss of the momentum around PHC (Schaay et al 2008).

However, the situation may be different in developed countries where in the US, for instance, some largely federally and locally funded health clinics are modernised with new equipment and electronic medical records. As the above example (Web 2012) demonstrates, in such countries there are likely to be space planning, design, and furniture installation for community health centre facilities that represents high costs in the community-investments that may include learning space designs that meet the needs of community health service and can accommodate many of the proposals in Table 35 for designing the learning environment to enhance learning in community.

Although development costs are high, costs for administering the programmes are low. As we have seen, advantages of ICTs include cost savings due to training being accessible to employees at their homes or offices and reduced costs associated with employees travelling to a central training location, for example, transport fare, food and lodging. Moreover, with the exception of distance learning, the most important characteristics needed for learning to occur (practice, feedback, etc) are built into these methods. Its effectiveness is likely to be high if the method including characteristics of a positive learning environment and learner control, sharing and linking are built into these methods. This is where the role of the educational technologist is important. The educational technologist understands how best technology is used in a particular space and can, among other things, advise on the type of technology that is needed. The issues surrounding development cost and the use of ICT to support cooperative and collaborative learning in the community are further discussed in following chapters.

There are useful considerations other than development costs for designing the learning environment in community health education, which relate to settings for community-based learning (Boaden et al 1999) and are relevant to the suggestions in Table 35. One is the professional orientation of the setting that may be exclusively medical or multi-faceted where medical professionals work with other professionals such as nurses, or the inclusion of non-professional practitioners like village health workers in the community health workforce. What is now clear, particularly in light of the needs of community health education, is that the professional exclusiveness that had characterised much of professional practice and education in the past must now change to a direction where different professional groups, including student groups, work together within the community. Macro-level theories suggest that, for example, employees are likely to feel more empowered to do their work in a more organically structured environment that supports clinical autonomy and collaborative professional relationships. Thus, designs of the learning environments should recognise this argument and must consider providing opportunities for collaborative working which is better suited to the present and future needs of community health education and practice. This issue is further discussed in the following chapters.

Another consideration for community health educators is the location of the learning environment to be designed. The scope of this may range from a large hospital to a local health facility, such as a health centre or clinic located in isolated areas, where health services are provided to a relatively smaller number of people. These local health facilities can serve as settings not only for community health practice, but also for research and education. However we have seen, for instance, that there are complexities in organisational arrangements and agency relationships within PHC organisation structures that are often problematic. For example, we have seen that there is promotion of vertical programmes by development partners like the Global Fund who, while providing much needed funding for priority diseases such as TB and AIDS, have simultaneously promoted the selective approach of PHC through privileging vertically implemented and managed programmes. Such programmes are often initiated at the central or tertiary level of PHC without the participation of local health officers in their planning. These programmes emphasise targets to be reached instead of building up systems that have the capacity to promote health and solve health problems, as well as facilitate learning in the community health centres and clinics. There are also the problems of geographic dispersion of trainees, trainees' difficulty in attending training, and whether new technologies are part of the health unit's business strategy.

An obvious need here is for community health educators and their collaborators to be clear about these differences in the locations where learning environments can be designed and the extent to which they interrelate and agree with the aim of designing learning environments that enhance community of learning and meet the requirements of community health education.

Some people think that illiteracy and geographic isolation of target groups serve as barriers to participation; however, with creativity and patience it is possible for community health educators and their partners to include the poorest, most isolated and illiterate of groups.This means that they must design learning environments that enhance the needed experiential learning that must include the participation of target groups in community health including its organisational structures, and make it possible for trainees to access such educational provisions. An important reason why society should care about learning in the community is that learning in a community will have an important part to play in preparing students for their work-life to come. These issues are further discussed in the following chapters, especially chapters dealing with professional development and development of teaching and learning centres.

Community health educators and their collaborators should consider the management style in the various community health agencies where learning environments are to be designed. We have already suggested that officials at the central level of PHC are inclined to use the bureaucratic management style in planning vertical programmes that fund and, consequently, influence community health education, especially professional development/continuing education programmes. This management style is characterised by clear division of labour, and levels of responsibilities and accountability. It contrasts very much with the democratic management style that is considered more appropriate at a local level (Collins et al 1994). The democratic management style is defined, for instance, by the manager working with community members to identify community health needs and needed policies and programmes. In this way, the healthcare manager is functioning as a leader and partner who includes the client at every step of the decision-making process of health care, thereby making the process of care more of a partnership approach. Thus, PHC teams that require such an approach to management should have more management capacity, as the role of the manager is to handle the many complex issues in the team. This includes understanding the different characteristics and modes of operations of the many agencies that provide settings for learning. This is required because such features will clearly influence the design of community health-centric learning environments. Again, these issues are further discussed in the following chapters, especially in the chapters dealing with professional development and development of teaching and learning centres.

Another factor that community health educators and their collaborators need to consider is the type of organisation. At the primary, secondary and tertiary levels of PHC are many non-governmental organisations (voluntary or private) providing both preventative and curative services in the rural and urban settings, in addition to the public health services. These different categories of service providers concern issues such as staff motivation, control, accountability that vary in the organisations (Boaden et al 1999). We have also seen that there may be difficulties concerning representation of local people. Attitudes and expectations, as we have seen in the foregoing discussion, may differ widely in community health agencies, but these difficulties have to be dealt with by community health education leaders in ways that result in mutual opportunities for designing learning environments.

Community health educators and their partners need to consider the related issue of patient/client accessibility to health services provided by public, private or voluntary health services. Here again there are variations in the factors that influence patient/client access - such as the kind of relationship between clients and service organisation, geography and the psychology of access (e.g. attitudes of health workers towards patients/clients), organisation, formal and informal rules of access, and location. Patient/client accessibility is necessary for the organisations to function effectively and is one of the major arguments for community-based organisations which are perceived as being more sensitive and accessible to patients and clients (ibid). The implication of this for community health education is that the kinds of interactions between trainees and others from the community that enhance community of learning are facilitated by increased accessibility by patients, clients and other community members to health facilities such as community health centres and clinics where community health education is provided. Community health educators must therefore take into account such factors to design the kinds of learning environments that enhance community of learning and community health–centric education. This leads to the final consideration.

The need for trainees to be aware of local communities, and to be able to work in and within such communities has been the subject of much debate and experimentation particularly in developing countries that have adopted the PHC approach (e.g. Richards 2001). This issue represents a major thrust of this book. There are at least two primary reasons why society should care about learning in community: (i) learning is a social process that works best in a community setting, thus yielding the best use of societal resources and (ii) teaching and learning in the community will have an important role to play in preparing students for their work-life to come. Graduates of professional training institutions, for example, must succeed in professional environments that require interactions with other people. Due to the volatility of information today and the increase of information flow, community-based education will help prepare graduates to live and work in a world that requires greater collaboration. The learning environment must be designed to provide opportunities for students to use effectively and continually what they have learned in their work in community health. This issue is especially central to the idea of building a community of learning in community health and is further discussed in the following chapters. Table 35 provides examples of activities that foster an engaged academic community.

**Table 35: Example of Activities that foster an engaged Academic Community**

**Pedagogical approaches that foster community.**

| Example | Implications for Learning Environment Design |
|---|---|
| Students experience a community-friendly learning environment from the beginning of the first class | Community-centric ambience of physical and virtual spaces should be readily discerned by faculty and students, from room lighting and decoration to learning management system usability |
| Faculty and students learn about each other and from each other | Mechanism for learning each other's names available in and out of the classroom. Students and instructor(s) post interests, photos, and backgrounds on course Web site. |
| Students participate in discussion in class. | Classroom "front" is deemphasized (removing the lectern, for example) to create open, discussion-friendly space. Choice and placement of furniture allows students to see and hear each other |
| Active learning activities in class use cooperative techniques. | Students are seated in proximity to each other but with flexibility for movement and space between chairs for instructor mobility. |
| Team-based projects are conducted outside class and culminate in student-led presentations. | Room technology enhancements and lighting controls should be immediately intuitive to student presenters. |
| In-class activities are augmented by completing a significant fraction of course expectations online | Courses use a learning management system that provides delivery of course materials online and enables exchange of messages, threaded discussions, announcements, homework assignments, quizzes, and grades |
| Classroom visitors, such as civic leaders or alumni, can broaden classroom community and enrich discussion | Rooms are easy for visitors to find and have extra seating and tables of adequate quality so as to send a positive image of the institution. Time in class can be used to make meaning out of the material rather than conduct "housekeeping" tasks |
| Video or telephone conference-based technologies enable discussion with experts in the field from inaccessible locations, such as overseas. | Conferencing equipment is placed in room, with remote or on-site technical management and setup |
| In-class integration of study skills and best practices nurture collaboration and improve student learning. | Space redesign should be connected to faculty development efforts that focus on learning-centered pedagogies. |
| Student-faculty interactions can occur immediately before and after a class | Broad pathways (not corridors) connect classrooms, with ample room for discussion and whiteboard use during class changes without impeding traffic flow |
| Students meet with faculty in office spaces that are easy to find and conducive to dialogue. | Building signage is clear and in keeping with universal design principles, to be accessible to all. Faculty office suites are large enough for meetings, with sufficient seating and board space |

**Cocurriculum that fosters community.**

| Example | Implications for Learning Environment Design |
|---|---|
| Orientation and preorientation events introduce students to the campus culture and help define standards of behavior and norms of civility. | Campus-wide architecture, landscaping, interior design, and even Web presence provide an ambience that immediately conveys openness, community, sociability, and safety. |
| Students live in residential housing closely associated, physically and culturally, with the campus. They can live together in thematic or curricular cohorts. | From campus master planning to student residential programming, housing should be integrated into a campus culture that sees the "living" part of a college education as linked to the academic experience. |
| Social and cultural activities explore and build on the institution's heritage, mission, and connection with alumni as well as the community. | A wide variety of physical spaces create places for campus involvement, including recreational and intramural sport facilities, religious and cultural gathering spaces, and a wide variety of formal and informal avenues for artistic representation. |
| Students participate in volunteer work to expand their understanding of social responsibilities and to develop leadership skills. | Meeting spaces and administrative centers house programs that develop student leadership and connect student clubs and organizations to service-learning opportunities. |
| Co-curricular activities involve students, faculty, and staff in shared dialogue. | Inviting, comfortable, and flexible spaces should be available for clubs and organizations so that more involved participation occurs with connections to academics, such as reading clubs to discuss popular books or hot topics. |
| Studying occurs anywhere and at any time. | Public and residential spaces, from the library to laundromats, can be made amenable to studying, including wireless network installation. Many factors such as safety, lighting, and noise control play into suitability for studying. |
| Students collaborate on team projects outside the classroom and participate in group study sessions. | Public areas such as dining and foyer spaces are considered social spaces. They are spacious, inviting, and accessible at times when students need to meet. |
| Students participate in experiential learning opportunities while on campus. | On-campus employment and student-run businesses should be created to expose students to a variety of relevant real-world business and administration learning experiences. |
| Students participate in campus management decisions to create a sense of ownership and responsibility. | Broaden student involvement in campus planning and administrative decision making, and respect their unique and critical viewpoint. |

*Source: Bickford et al 2010*

## Summary

The chapter has looked at how community health educators and their partners can be involved in designing learning spaces in community health. To undertake new learning space building projects in the community, community health educators and their partners should identify the overall goals and stakeholders as early as possible; obtain the support and agreement of the highest possible institutional leaders in their organisations; identify and develop all possible funding sources and supporters as early as possible;  involve educational technologists, who can provide on-the-ground support to faculty members and learners and therefore can check existing and new technologies; and involve information technologists, who are essential in developing an appropriate ICT infrastructure, data management plan, support services and adaptability to support the learning technologies designed for learning space. They must bring their facility planning and project management team, which may include key stakeholders from universities such as educational technologists into the process at the earliest stages so they can assist in the creation of a project structure and organisation, task lists, conceptual schedules and project budget estimates, etc. The following chapter further deals with the important issue of technology, community and information exchange in relation to building a community of learning in community health.

# 9

## Technology, Community, and Information Exchange

As already discussed, there are significant advances in community health and the education of health professionals in community health that demand the creation and support of more diverse and complex technology in learning spaces in the community than ever before. The education of health professionals for community health is increasingly moving beyond planning for instruction in on-campus facilities and resources to greater use of new learning spaces with ICTs for learning (e.g Intel World Ahead programme 2010).

We have seen that there is now a growing interest by health educationists and other stakeholders in ICTs because of the positive educational outcomes that can result from the use of ICTs in education. The educational technologist's role in the learning space design process, as indicated, is important for several reasons, such as the educational technologist having deep understanding of how technology is used in a particular space and can assist community health educators select the proper type of technology.

All these help to integrate the appropriate technology infrastructure to help ensure a successful outcome of the learning space design. Also, as mentioned, technology decisions affect space design while space design effects specific technology decisions. This is why, as we have seen, decisions on ICTs must accompany the learning space design which strongly influences the ease with which ICTs are integrated by means of, for example:

- the relationships and commitment established with partners and local people, particularly the intended primary stakeholders
- the logic and feasibility of the ICT planning strategy
- the resources allocated to ICT plans (funding, time, expertise)
- the degree of in-built flexibility that allows ICT plans to have an operational function

- any operational details of the ICT plans that might be established during initial design

This chapter will consider issues relating to the appropriateness of ICTs and their use to further a community of learning in community health. A discussion of new technologies that influence community health education delivery will be provided, followed by a review of the considerations for choosing appropriate ICTs for enhancing cooperative and collaborative learning which, as already mentioned, serves as the principal means of fostering community of learning in community health education. Finally, the chapter describes several types of ICT tools that can be used in synchronous and asynchronous learning for this purpose.

## How New Technologies Are Influencing Community Health Higher Education

In higher education, communication is playing a critical role in building and sustaining a community of learners. ICT solutions offer an outstanding arena for connecting and sharing information among community members in or outside the classroom. Questions of when and where learning occurs can be addressed by ICTs which is broadening the scope of planning for new or renovated physical spaces. At one end, physical learning spaces may no longer be necessary if an academic programme is delivered online, while at the other end, face-to-face classes can happen in various physical spaces that take advantage of technology in or out of the space (Bickford et al 2010).

In these learning situations or contexts, technology should be used to foster learning through building community as well as creating and sharing knowledge within the group while allowing interaction to take place in and outside the formal classroom setting. There are several ways ICTs can foster a community of learning: (1) in particular, communication outside the classroom can become richer and more extensive using tools such as threaded discussions, e-mail and instant messaging (2) ICTs can be used to build student understanding outside the classroom and free classroom time for more active pedagogical approaches (ibid). By using ICT solutions to share course content outside scheduled class time, faculty can use the face-to-face time in the classroom for more active learning approaches.

This, as seen in the previous chapter (Table 35), requires among other things, designing classrooms with much greater flexibility for various pedagogical approaches. The use of mobile computing for students is being considered or implemented by many institutions (ibid). Students can research or write papers while networking to build community using such a device. Since learning occurs in a variety of spaces, mobility and academic requirements for technology access are important arguments, as learning happens in various places.

ICTs are also gaining popularity in healthcare education worldwide and innovations in medical education, for example, include further application of ICTs and academic web-casting (Trucano 2005). In resource-limited countries, in particular, setting up of an academic web-casting programmes could facilitate curricular, adopt more student-centred learning applications, enrich students' learning experiences, enhance trainer-trainee collaboration and provide evidence-based practice material. It might also add to reducing the effects of shortage of teaching faculty (ibid). With ICTs and the academic web-casting, educators in these countries can also increase enrolment, because the open ICT can deliver a lecture to thousands of students. For most health educational institutions worldwide, the Information Age has ushered in a variety of technology innovations that are fundamentally changing the quality of healthcare delivery and education. ICTs have become essential commodities within the modern healthcare system – as important as the books and medical equipment or pharmaceuticals. ICTs are part of continuing education to physicians, nurses and other students who are increasingly becoming reliant on the Internet and other online resources to keep up-to-date with current educational literature.

Thus, the importance now placed on ICTs in community health education is increasing and this is likely to intensify in the 21st century. Therefore, it is necessary to look at important considerations in making technology decisions that can influence community health education now and in the future.

### Considerations for Choosing ICTs to enhance Information Exchange in Community Health Education

Technology decisions that affect community health education must include making sound judgment on the appropriate use of technology for community health education as required by the PHC approach to health care. One of the principles of the PHC approach - the basis on which community health in mainly developing countries context is implemented - is appropriate technology. The PHC principle of appropriate technology helps community health educators make sound decisions on the choice of ICTs for enhancing community of learning in community health education. The aim must be to use ICTs that are most appropriate for furthering this process in both developed and developing countries. As Trucano (ibid) commented, generally technology changes rapidly and newer, more cost-effective and more powerful technologies will continue to emerge for potential use in education. At the same time, according to Trucano (ibid), evidence shows that, once installed in schools, ICTs continue to be used for the duration of the functioning life of the technology, whether or not newer, more cost-effective and powerful technologies emerge. Trucano (ibid) also says that much of the publicly available information about the effectiveness of particular ICT tools is generated by the companies who market such products and related services, which further makes it necessary for the choice of technology to be given careful thought.

In making decisions on the choice of ICT tools for enhancing a community of learning for community health education, we also need to further narrow and focus the choice of ICT tools. This is due to the rapidly changing nature of ICTs and the different conceptions on learning that influence the choice of technology, among other things. To do this, we must return to an earlier discussion in Part One, Chapter 5 on collaborative learning. As mentioned there, the collaborative learning mode is arguably not only more definable than the other modes of learning that enhance community of learning it is also more useful for meeting the educational requirements of community health and the community of learning idea. Collaborative learning is aimed at getting the students to take almost full responsibility for working together, changing and evolving together, and of course building knowledge together.

The learning process is defined by what the learner does by activating already existing cognitive structures or by constructing new cognitive structures that receive new input (Dooly 2008). Rather than the learner passively receiving knowledge from the teacher; teaching becomes a transaction between all stakeholders (ibid). Using this approach for learning in the community, students can engage in many activities to form the social interactions needed to establish and build community of learning in community health. They can create a community in the absence of important faculty involvement. Also, by using this framework, faculty can have a positive impact on shaping, contributing to, and extending the learning environment of students in the community. However, the teacher should remember that the best method for exchanging information and opinions, as well as the choice of ICTs for doing this, rests on several contextual factors, such as the objectives of the overall project, age of students, the group personality and local constraints.

Therefore, due to the newness of e-learning, there is need for sharing experiences in e-learning across national borders as ICT is growing daily in the developing world, such as in Africa where perhaps this need is more important to consider than in the developed world. Trucano (2005), for instance, presents a Knowledge Map on ICT in education in developing countries with these guiding questions: (1) What is known about which ICTs are most useful to benefit education? (2) What do we know about the usefulness, appropriateness and efficacy of specific ICTs (including radio, television, handheld devices, computers, networked computers and the Internet) for educational purposes? (3) What do we know about the use of open source and free software in education?

On the basis of these guiding queries (ibid) found that the Internet is not widely available in least developed countries (LDCs); broadcast technologies such as radio and television have a much greater penetration than the Internet throughout much of the developing world. This substantial gap is not expected to be closed soon. Although educational initiatives that utilise radio and television typically have quite high initial start-up/capital costs, ongoing maintenance and upgrade costs are much lower (making initiatives utilising radio and TV for distance learning in the education sector particularly appealing for donor support in many cases) (ibid). One-to-many broadcast technologies like radio and television (as well as satellite distribution of electronic content) are perceived as being less 'revolutionary' ICTs in education, because their use is seen as reinforcing traditional instructor-centric learning models (Trucano ibid). Contrarily, computers are often seen as important tools in fostering more learner-centric instructional (ibid).

As well as being well studied, radio instruction has been utilised broadly. Especially, studies on radio instruction have focused on the links between the use of radio in combination with school-based educational resources and a variety of pedagogical practices (ibid). The results of projects on the use of TV in a few places have shown success in reaching out-of-school youth in a number of countries, especially in Latin America and China (ibid). Market liberalisation in some cases have enabled ICTs (like radio and the Internet, and to a lesser extent television) to be used to distribute educational content regionally within a country. Such educational content is more targeted to the needs of specific communities. Because of this they have a greater flexibility to employ local languages.

Computer-aided instruction (CAI) still receives much interest in LDCs. Computers are seen as simple replacements for teachers and have been largely discredited, although there appears to still be great interest in CAI in many LDCs where computers are being introduced (ibid). There is the issue of where to store computers, as it is unclear where to put computers to ensure they are utilised most efficiently. Research on the most appropriate placement of computers in schools, or in the community, used to achieve various learning objectives seems limited.

Likewise, Multi-Channel Learning (MCL) is seen as a useful technique. Its emerging practice concentrates on enriching the educational experience by engaging all resources that are available to help effect incremental change by coordinating the various ways to connect learners with information, knowledge, and stimulation, and to mediate those interactions (ibid). Also, MCL provides valuable insight into how blended learning approaches can be delivered and tailored in areas of great resource scarcity (ibid).

Not the same can be said about satellite which is much hyped, but under-studied. Although thought to have much promise, satellite broadcasting of electronic educational resources has not been studied enough to show if it can be used successfully in LDCs.

Similarly, New Internet Technologies hold promise, but are not yet operational. New Internet technologies, particularly recent and emerging wireless protocols (including 802.11, and shortly WiMax), while thought to hold much promise for providing connectivity to remote areas, projects utilising such technologies are for the most part in pilot or planning stages, and face many regulatory hurdles ( ibid).

To reach rural areas, Mobile Internet centres (vans, etc.) are being deployed to such areas, and quite a number of educational initiatives using mobile Internet centres have been piloted in the past decade (ibid). However, cost and impact data from such projects have been scarce.

Community telecentres (sometimes based in schools) have been commended as important tools to provide access to learners (including teachers engaged in personal enrichment and professional development opportunities) to ICTs outside of formal school settings (ibid). However, replicable models have yet to emerge.

Limited research has been conducted on uses of handheld devices (including personal digital assistants and mobile phones) in education, which is just now receiving serious widespread attention.

Likewise, 'Free software' (which grants the user the right to run the software, inspect, modify, and distribute the source-code/software) holds promise, but costs and impact are still not well documented. The uses of 'free' software (for example, GNU/Linux, Apache and LibreOffice) are widely commended as a cost effective alternative to the uses of proprietary software (especially Microsoft products) (ibid). However, research in this area is mainly advocatory in character. For example, the Asmoz Foundation, under the Department of Industry, Innovation, Commerce and Tourism of the Basque Government, has carried out a project called "RESEARCH AND PROMOTION OF FREE SOFTWARE TECHNOLOGY PLATFORMS FOR MASSIVE OPEN ONLINE COURSES" (Sanzberro et al 2014) with the aim of examining the trend in e-Learning from a technological perspective and in collaboration with the UPV/EHU (University of the Basque Country), with a view to contributing towards its establishment as a valid model for permanent education in the Basque Autonomous Community. The conclusions reached will be published and disseminated to universities, schools, education agents and companies. Box 13 shows the results of the project which demonstrate its supportive nature.

**Box 13: Results of the Project on Research and Promotion of Free Software Technology Platforms for Massive Open Online Courses**

In general, the results obtained through the project have been

- To research and test the different open source online learning platforms that enable the provision of Massive Open Online Courses (MOOC)-style education.
- To give teachers (indispensable vector) the opportunity to generate 'massive open online courses' by themselves, as this group has few conceptual and pragmatic references that suggest how to approach the work from this new perspective.
- To promote the implementation of this new trend in education among teachers, leading to education free of charge provided by platforms that are accessible through the Internet and focused on very large groups of people. MOOCs are usually based on up-to-date material, are focused on practical aspects and have a curriculum that depends on the interests of the pupils.
- To study the problems and technological needs that arise when defining and developing MOOCs.
- To disseminate the study carried out throughout the education community (Universities, schools, education agents and companies) and to provide solutions to the extent possible.

*Source: Sanzberro et al (2014)*

Currently, there appears to be more data related to the potential benefits of free software in education. For example, Terbuc (2014) indicates that free software is available and well-established, and that the possibility of choosing and using free software and didactic applications by teachers and students in the teaching process has increased. Terbuc (2014) cites the results of a study by Tonga (2004) on the use of free software in education which he says corresponds with his own findings. These results show that:

- Free software can lower the barriers to the access of ICTs by reducing the cost of software
- It is better in terms of performance, reliability and security
- There is increasing need of governments, industry and other organisations for graduates familiar with free software technology
- The open philosophy of free software is consistent with open dissemination of knowledge, information sharing in academia and academic freedom
- Use of free software discourages piracy by students, who often cannot afford the cost of licensed copies of the propriety software. If students are unable to access free software they are likely to use illegal copies of propriety software to do their work

- Free software can be localised because one can access the source code, which may not be possible with propriety software whose source code is seldom released for users to study.

What has been said so far about making decisions on ICTs for education highlights the difficulties that community health educators and their partners who engage in such decision-making face. However, these challenges can provide opportunities for debate between the different stakeholders in the building process that can produce positive outcomes. We have seen that the educational technologist's role in the learning space design process can include providing deep understanding of how technology is used in a particular space and can give useful advice on the type of technology to be selected, etc. Also, we have seen that the educator's task as a member of the design team is to ensure that decisions are made that result in a physical environment joined with current and future needs for learning and/or assessment. As already indicated, cognitive collaboration/co-operation, for example, becomes operational when two or more learners work interactively building a joint solution to a problem. What are the kinds of ICTs that can be used to enhance cooperative and collaborative learning in community health education? Concentrating on the cooperative and collaborative modes of learning helps to further narrow and focus the choice of ICTs. The following section presents several ICTs that can facilitate information exchange in community health education within the synchronous and asynchronous learning frameworks that complement cooperative/collaborative learning in the education process.

## Types of ICT Tools that can Facilitate Information Exchange in Community Health Education

As we have seen in Part One, Chapter 5, information exchange plays a critical role in social interactions and contributes significantly to facilitating learning and improving student engagement through community. We have also seen that network-based learning is a good way to design tasks that include ways of giving students the chance to analyse, synthesise, and evaluate their ideas together in groups in keeping with particularly the collaborative mode of learning. As indicated, these higher order thinking skills which serve as means of facilitating discussion and interaction that encourage students to progress beyond mere statements of opinion are learnt synchronously or asynchronously. Thus, the synchronous and asynchronous learning modes which complement cooperative/collaborative learning in the educational process can provide the needed approaches for information exchange in the community.

Although the synchronous and asynchronous learning modes are the two primary forms of online learning modalities, both forms of learning have positive and negative aspects, and strategies for facilitating their learning also differ. The roles of the facilitator and the student are characterised by the methods of academic delivery. The following sections present a detailed view (Kaplan et al 2003) of some of the synchronous and asynchronous communication tools that can be used by community health schools to create a full, rich learning experience and sense of community for their students. In the next chapter on pedagogy, curricular and co-curricular design, we will explore and compare the differences between asynchronous and synchronous learning facilitation strategies, facilitation and learner roles, and delivery within a synchronous and asynchronous learning environment.

**Synchronous Tools**

Synchronous tools enable real-time communication and collaboration in a "same time-different place" mode. These tools allow people to connect at a single point in time, at the same time. Synchronous tools possess the advantage of being able to engage people instantly and at the same point in time. The primary drawback of synchronous tools is that, by definition, they require same-time participation - different time zones and conflicting schedules can create communication challenges. In addition, they tend to be costly and may require significant bandwidth to be efficient (Kaplan et al 2003). Table 36 presents advantages and limitations of synchronous tools.

**Table 36: Synchronous Tools**

| Tool | Description | Useful for | Limitations |
|---|---|---|---|
| Audio conferencing | A conference call is a telephone call in which the calling party wishes to have more than one called party listen in to the audio portion of the call. | Discussions and dialogue | Costly, especially when international participation is involved |
| Web conferencing | Web conferencing refers to a service that allows conferencing events to be shared with remote locations. These are sometimes referred to as webinars or, for interactive conferences, online workshops | Sharing presentations and information | Cost, bandwidth; may also require audio conferencing to be useful |
| Video conferencing | Videoconferencing is the conduct of a videoconference by a set of telecommunication technologies which allow two or more locations to communicate by simultaneous two-way video and audio transmissions. It has also been called 'visual collaboration' and is a type of groupware. | In-depth discussions with higher-touch interactions | Cost, limited availability of video conferencing systems |

| | | | |
|---|---|---|---|
| Chat | On the Internet, chatting is talking to other people who are using the Internet at the same time you are. Usually, this "talking" is the exchange of typed-in messages requiring one site as the repository for the messages (or "chat site") and a group of users who take part from anywhere on the Internet. In some cases, a private chat can be arranged between two parties who meet initially in a group chat. Chats can be ongoing or scheduled for a particular time and duration. | Information sharing of low-complexity issues | Usually requires typing, "lower touch" experience |
| Instant messaging | Instant messaging (IM) is a type of online chat which offers real-time text transmission over the Internet | Ad hoc quick communications | All users must use compatible system, usually best for 1:1 interactions |
| White boarding | A term used to describe the placement of shared documents on an on-screen whiteboard. Desktop videoconferencing software includes "snapshot" tools that enable one to capture entire windows or portions of windows and place them on the whiteboard. | Co-development of ideas | Cost, bandwidth; may also require audio conferencing to be useful |
| Application s | Application sharing is an element of remote access, falling under the collaborative software umbrella that enables two or more users to access a shared application or document from their respective computers simultaneously in real time. | Co-development of documents | Cost, bandwidth; may also require audio conferencing to be useful |

**Source: Adapted from Kaplan et al (2003)**

**Asynchronous Tools**

Asynchronous tools enable communication and collaboration over a period of time through a "different time-different place" mode. These tools allow people to connect together at each person's own convenience and own schedule. Asynchronous tools are useful for sustaining dialogue and collaboration over a period of time and providing people with resources and information that are instantly accessible, day or night. Asynchronous tools possess the advantage of being able to involve people from multiple time zones. In addition, asynchronous tools are helpful in capturing the history of the interactions of a group, allowing for collective knowledge to be more easily shared and distributed. The primary drawback of asynchronous technologies is that they require some discipline to use when used for ongoing communities of practice (e.g. people typically must take the initiative to "login" to participate) and they may feel "impersonal" to those who prefer higher-touch synchronous technologies (Kaplan et al 2003). Table 37 indicates advantages and limitations of asynchronous tools.

**Table 37: Asynchronous Tools**

| Tool | Description | Useful for | Limitations |
|---|---|---|---|
| Discussion boards | Any online "bulletin board" where you can leave and expect to see responses to messages you have left. Or you can just read the board. | Dialogue that takes place over a period of time | May take longer to arrive at decisions or conclusions |
| Web logs (Blogs) | Weblog is a form of communication and publishing on the Internet | Sharing ideas and comments | May take longer to arrive at decisions or conclusions |
| Messaging (e-mail) | Messaging (also called electronic messaging ) is the creation, storage, exchange, and management of text, images, voice, telex, fax , e-mail, paging, and Electronic Data Interchange ( EDI ) over a communications network | One-to-one or one-to-many communications | May be misused as a "collaboration tool" and become overwhelming |

| | | | |
|---|---|---|---|
| Streaming audio | Streaming audio is multimedia that is constantly received by and presented to an end-user while being delivered by a provider | Communicating or teaching | Static and typically does not provide option to answer questions or expand on ideas |
| Streaming video | Streaming video is content sent in compressed form over the Internet and displayed by the viewer in real time | Communicating or teaching | Static and typically does not provide option to answer questions or expand on ideas |
| Narrated slideshows | Narrated slideshows include audio recordings synchronised to images without hand-drawn annotations. | Communicating or teaching | Static and typically does not provide option to answer questions or expand on ideas |
| "Learning objects" (Web-based training) | Web-based training (sometimes called e-learning) is anywhere, any-time instruction delivered over the Internet or Intranet to browser-equipped learners | Teaching and training | Typically does not provide option to answer questions or expand on ideas in detail |
| Database | A collection of information organied in such a way that a computer programme can quickly select desired pieces of data. You can think of a database as an electronic filing system. | Managing information and knowledge | Requires clear definition and skillful administration |
| Web books | A webbook is a portmanteau of web and notebook computer, and is a generic class of laptop computers such as the litl, Elonex and Coxion webbook computers. | Teaching and training | Not dynamic and may lose interest of users |

| | | | |
|---|---|---|---|
| Surveys and polls | A poll allows you to ask one multiple choice question. Participants can choose from among answers that you predefine. You can allow the voter to select just one answer or allow them to choose multiple answers. You also have the option of adding another field to allow a voter to enter their own answer. A survey, in contrast, allows you to ask multiple questions across a wider range of question types. So you can ask for a comment, an email address, a name, an address etc., as well as multiple choice questions. | Capturing information and trends | Requires clear definition and ongoing coordination |
| Shared Calendars | Sharing is the ability to grant another user access to one or more of your calendars. For example:<br>• You can give a coworker view permission to a project calendar that you maintain. In this case, your coworker will see your shared calendar in his or her own Calendar view. Whenever you schedule an appointment or meeting on the shared calendar, your coworker will see the appointment or meeting.<br>• You can also give a coworker Manager permission to your account. In this case, your coworker will be able to do the following with the shared calendar:<br>• View meetings and appointments<br>• Schedule meetings and appointments<br>• Accept and decline meeting invitations<br>• Edit and delete meetings and appointments | Coordinating activities | System compatibility |

| | | | |
|---|---|---|---|
| Web site links | A link to a website is a spot on a Web page that, when clicked, takes the visitor to the Web address (URL) specified in the link definition. This link can be in the form of text or a graphic, either of which the visitor clicks to go to the other site. | Providing resources and referenc-es | May become outdated and "broken" |

*Adapted from Kaplan et al (2003)*

A significant step beyond this appetiser of individual tools are web-based platforms that aim to provide some or most of the functionality of these stand-alone tools, but do so within a single integrated collaborative environment. The integration and synthesis of these tools creates a container that turns out to be far greater than the sum of its parts and can become the single portal for all community activities. Going beyond mixing together these items in a disordered mass of individual technologies can elevate students' experiences by encouraging collaborative learning and knowledge sharing (ibid).

Students should explore the differences between asynchronous and synchronous learning prior to choosing a mode of academic interaction. Reviewing the advantages and disadvantages, facilitation strategies, facilitator and student roles, and delivery methods will provide students with enough information to make an educated decision about the best path for him or her. Online facilitators should follow the same procedure to determine which method of teaching is preferred. Here again, the roles of community health educators, educational technologists, information technologists and facilities managers, especially the educational technologist, are crucial, for he/she better understands how technology is used in a particular space and can advise on the type of technology that should be selected, the physical placement of equipment in the space, and the user interfaces that need to be designed to make the technology easy to use in various community learning settings including health centres and clinics. These issues are further discussed in following chapters.

**Summary**

This chapter has considered issues relating to the appropriateness of ICTs and their use to further community of learning in community health. It began by discussing how new technologies influence community health education delivery. After this, the chapter presented considerations for choosing appropriate ICTs for enhancing cooperative and collaborative learning. Finally, the chapter described several types of ICTs that can be used in synchronous and asynchronous learning to support cooperative and collaborative learning, including audio conferencing, web conferencing, video conferencing, chat, instant messaging, white boarding and application sharing. This is to exemplify how technology can be used to support cooperative and collaborative learning through serving as a storage place for intellectual capital information and learned capabilities. The chapter then outlined the usefulness of the tools as well as their limitations.

The next chapter considers pedagogy, curricular and co-curricular design which includes an exploration and comparison of the differences between asynchronous and synchronous learning facilitation strategies, facilitation and learner roles, and delivery within a synchronous and asynchronous learning environment.

# 10

## *Pedagogical, Curricular, and Co-curricular Design*

The pedagogy education theory provides the teacher with the principal responsibility of deciding content of learning, learning method and evaluation (Knowles, as cited by Noe 1999). Generally, students are perceived as being passive recipients of direction and content, and coming with little experience that can be a useful resource to the teaching and learning environment (ibid). Androgogy, the theory of adult learning, was developed as a reaction to such shortcomings of formal education theories, with these assumptions: adults have a need to be self-directed, adults have the need to know why they are learning something, adults are motivated to learn by intrinsic as well as extrinsic factors. Additionally, adults enter into a learning experience with a problem-centred approach to learning, and bring more work-related experiences into the learning environment. This theory is particularly significant to think of when designing environments that foster a community of learning in community health for many of the students are usually adults.

Co-curriculum refers to educational activities that are complementary but are not part of the regular curriculum. (refer to Chapter 3 for definitions of the curriculum). Co-curriculum is modelled on development theories which suggest that students move from a rather insular view of themselves and the world (e.g. Ahmed 2011). As a result of their experiences and learning which occurs both in-and out-of the classroom they develop into individuals with a more defined identity and pluralistic view of the world. Specifically, as students move along this continuum of cognitive and personal development, they develop a sense of purpose where they are able to formulate personal, intellectual, and career goals, develop competence and experience growth in their intellectual, interpersonal, and physical skills, develop their personal identity by becoming aware of their gender, sexual orientation, self-acceptance, and self-esteem (e.g. Ahmed 2011).

How can designers of pedagogical, curricular and co-curricular plans ensure that all these conditions are present in training programmes that foster a community of learning in community health? This chapter discusses features of effective curriculum design that incorporate these characteristics and elements for building a community of learning, offering examples and conceptual interpretations based on training programmes and frameworks for building a community of learning drawn from the education, management and community health literature. First, the chapter looks briefly at the curriculum design process, including how to choose curriculum models that facilitate a community of learning in community health education and giving a multiple curricular approach that agrees with the pedagogical, curricular and co-curricular design process. Finally, the chapter outlines the designing of student and faculty pedagogical, curricular and co-curricular activities in the community with emphasis on the use of the cooperative and collaborative learning modes, as well as the complementary synchronous and asynchronous learning techniques.

**Design Process**

Developing pedagogical, curricular, and co-curricular plans should also parallel the learning space design which strongly influences the ease with which pedagogical, curricular, and co-curricular plans are implemented later on through, for example:

- the relationships and commitment established with partners and local people, particularly the intended primary stakeholders
- the logic and feasibility of the design strategy
- the resources allocated to pedagogical, curricular, and co-curricular plans (funding, time, expertise)
- the degree of in-built flexibility that allows pedagogical, curricular, and co-curricular plans to have an operational function
- any operational details of the pedagogical, curricular, and co-curricular plans that might be established during initial design

As part of the pedagogical, curricular, and co-curricular design process, a broad pedagogical, curricular, and co-curricular framework should be developed to provide: (a) sufficient detail to enable budgeting and allocation of technical expertise (b) an overview of how pedagogical, curricular, and co-curricular plans will be implemented, and (c) some guidance for all involved about how pedagogical, curricular, and co-curricular plans should be developed (e.g. Flinders University 2013). Much of what is developed for the pedagogical, curricular, and co-curricular component during the learning space design stage will only be indicative of the final plan and will need to be revised and refined during implementation.

As we mentioned in Part Two, Chapter 8, the educator who will ultimately use the learning space must be an integral member of the learning space design team. The educator's task as a member of the design team is to ensure that decisions are made that result in a physical environment joined with current and future needs for learning and/or assessment by effectively communicating major components to the design team, such as education trends (e.g. flexibility, interactivity, learning strategies like team-based learning or cooperative/collaborative learning), customer needs (e.g. internet access, faculty development of users), and health technology (e.g. telemedicine). For example, in such a participatory process of curriculum development in community health (Tenn et al 1994) the actual development of the curriculum itself was undertaken by a core-group consisting of the coordinator of the course, public health nursing supervisors, the education consultant and public health nurses. The core group was guided and advised concerning curriculum development by an advisory committee made up of 15 health personnel: educators, nursing administrators, medical officers, health inspectors, health educators, and health statistics and planning personnel.

The main function of the advisory committee was to communicate divergent views, to make sure that the programme was relevant, making decisions on issues on which there were disagreements, granting the right to reject suggestions, and lobbying for acceptance of the programme at the development stage. At the evaluation stage, a renewed advisory committee, consisting mainly of nurses, served as the channel through which the process was approved and data findings renewed.

Nurses (professionals) involvement was ensured by including at different stages in the development and evaluation process practising nurses in healthcare settings in urban and rural areas who, on the basis of their practical experience, were able to identify numerous learning needs. They were able to provide the realities of public/community health practice and give information about the relevance of the programme and their expectations in terms of public/community health practice. They also provided data regarding the implementation of the programme.

The development of such a broad pedagogical, curricular, and co-curricular framework must consider the characteristics and environment of what is to be learnt. Thus, the primary focus of the curriculum design should be on the socio-economic model for self-reliance (Part One, Chapter 7) in health. As already indicated, the concept of self-reliance is located centrally within the discourse of community development and is connected to related concepts like self-help, mutual-help, indigenous participation and rural development. Self-help, for example, enables local people to make use of their under-utilised labour by exploiting to their advantage resources that would otherwise lie dormant. That way, they are able to deal with the twin challenges of ignorance and poverty of their communities.

Self-help for community development increases the competence and confidence of a community in handling its affairs. The habit of self-help is a prerequisite for survival in the modern world (e.g. Galtong et al, as cited by Fonchingong et al 2003). Self-help initiatives enable people to look inwards by rallying local resources and efforts. This is especially relevant to the concept of community development, which stresses the importance of people increasing their sense of responsibility, and considering assistance as just supplementary, but never replacing popular initiatives or local efforts. The emphasis is on democratising with reliance on what people can do for themselves. The principle of self-help incorporates into the community development process the means of offering ordinary citizens the opportunity to share in making important decisions about their living conditions. This approach echoes the people-centredness of community development-attempts at satisfying felt needs. This entails community participation at all levels of the development intervention. The self-reliance concept advocates the need for people to improve their condition using local initiatives and resources in their own hands (Fonchingong et al 2003).

In designing pedagogical, curricular, and co-curricular plans such a curriculum development team identifies the elements of the curriculum, states what their relationships are to one another and indicates the principles of organisation and the requirements of that organisation for the administrative conditions under which it is to operate. Such a design needs to be supported by a curriculum theory or theories/models which create the sources to consider and the principles to apply.

**Selecting Curriculum Models**

As we mentioned in Part 1, Chapter 3, the task of creating new courses of study or new patterns of educational activity for students demands curriculum design. As we have seen, there are many factors that are involved in the design of such intended curricula, such as ideological, technical, epistemological, and psychological. A systematic approach to developing curricular that considers these factors, compared to piecemeal, one-off modifications to current practice, is still relatively new and in consequence is both tentative and primitive. Also, as already mentioned, several curriculum design models have been produced to advance the business of designing curricular. Therefore, it is necessary to select the kinds of curriculum models that can include all the conditions, concepts and principles covered in Part 1 to be used in pedagogical, curricular and co-curricular design to build a community of learning in community health and through which the conceptions of education in particular can be given tangible form as curriculum proposals for the building of a community of learning process.

We saw in Part One, Chapter 3, that the objectives model (and similar prescriptive curriculum models we have looked at) is deemed insufficient for meeting these educational requirements, because it is philosophically and psychologically not that practical and humanistic for education (Lawton 1983) including community health education. The model can only be used for particular kinds of low-level skills and not the entire community-oriented curriculum. The objective model is that of a close system, whereas in a democratic society individuals need to be autonomous through an open-ended curriculum, which is the hallmark of the descriptive curriculum models outlined above. They are the process model, the situational analysis model and the cultural analysis model, which view curriculum work as a complex human activity. It is grounded in the complexity of practice, and describes what actually happens in a conceptual way. However, such descriptive models that are more comprehensive and open-ended can be employed together with objectives (used in a restricted way) to provide a complex and multifaceted approach to curriculum planning that is much preferred to single model strategies.

As discussed, an effort to solve the problem of objectives came as a proposal that each aspect of the curriculum should be examined separately on the premise that various curricula activities or subject areas will need different curriculum planning approaches. As a result of this, some writers have proposed a different type of separation of curriculum activities that can be justified educationally from those that are instrumental, and kinds of training for which statements of intent are not only acceptable but even necessary (e.g. Stenhouse 1975). This eclectic approach is arguably a proper and acceptable approach to planning pedagogical, curricular and co-curricular activities for students in building a community of learning in community health.

Also, as discussed, the advantages and disadvantages of the subject-centred, objectives and process models in Part One, Chapter 3, can apply to Beattie's four fold model as it includes the features of these models in its framework. However, there are two shortcomings of the models that have been suggested by Quinn (1995) that must be looked at. One shortcoming is that all the models, with the exception of Beattie's model, have all been formulated for the education of children; that the educational ideologies on which they are based are tenets of childhood education. Another imperfection is the failure of all the models, including Beattie's model, to consider the requirements and opinions of service managers/employers on the outputs they need for education and training to meet their service contracts. We have however noted that a significant external issue in the situational analysis model that curriculum planners should ask about is the expectations of employers. These issues should be dealt with by training administration.

As mentioned in Chapter 4 there are several suggestions on the learning process for the design of instruction. One of these is that students need the educational programme to be well arranged and coordinated. This is one of the many components of the responsibilities of those administering the educational programme. This requirement entails activities such as communicating courses and programmes to students and enrolling students in courses and programmes. But perhaps most importantly, as a requirement for building a community of learning, the responsibilities of the leader in the pedagogy, curricular and co-curricular design process must include ensuring that students are not distracted by events that could interfere with learning, such as the roadblocks we considered in Part One, Chapter 7. Using this multiple curricular approach enables a community health educators and their partners to incorporate many of the pedagogical, curricular and co-curricular activities that can foster a community of learning that Table 35 demonstrates, including in particular cooperative and collaborative learning.

As mentioned, the curriculum models we have considered above do not describe how curricula are in fact designed, rather they present different ideas on how the teaching and learning /planning task should be carried out, which is the subject of the following sections. We begin with a look at two examples from community-based medical education, relating the teacher and student activities to the curricular proposals we outlined above.

**Students and Faculty Activities in the Community**

Students can engage in many activities to form the social interactions needed to establish and build a community. For example, they can create a community in the absence of important faculty involvement (Bickford et al 2010). Thus, it is sensible to coordinate and improve pedagogical approaches, the curriculum, and the co-curricular experiences of students with the goal of creating a community that is friendlier to learners and is distinguished by participation.

Also, as already mentioned, in the curriculum design process planners should consider the possibility of using an eclectic approach including applying the curriculum model that is based on subjects. There are at least two reasons why using this curriculum model is so important: maintaining the self–confidence of subject-specialist teachers and the need for community health schools to be concerned with public or professional knowledge, which is usually organised in subjects or disciplines. For example, Eraut (1994) has identified and classified three kinds of knowledge that underpin professional education, which Boaden et al (1999) discuss using examples of teaching methods in the community drawn from the literature.

The first type of professional knowledge is propositional knowledge. This is connected to the discipline-based concepts, principles and generalisations that define general practice and that can be used in professional activities (Boaden et al 1999). The nature of propositional knowledge associated with community-based education refers to the content of the discipline such as epidemiology, statistics, decision-making, health care, economics, ethics, computer science etc. These elements are additional to the "core" of, for example, medicine (anatomy, biochemistry, physiology, etc) and are necessary for the effective practice of the discipline in the broader community-oriented health service. Such a "core" curriculum consists of a group of essential courses embodying the fundamentals of medicine generally, or specifically, of community-oriented health care, and it is given to students "before more individualised opportunities for focused study are presented". These components feed into the major areas of community health practice such as disease prevention, environmental health and health care organisation components which conventionally contained them (Boaden et al 1999). Therefore, the use of subjects in planning such a curriculum may be justifiable and necessary for including critical content in the curriculum concerning the eight elements of PHC/ community health.

While the important link between propositional knowledge and community-based education cannot be denied, it is the manner in which students learn such core-knowledge that has to change if it is to be of much use (Boaden et al 1999). Curriculum planners must consider ways by which students can use propositional knowledge through the higher order thinking skills of replication (the process of repeating what has been learnt), application (using knowledge in new situations), interpretation (bringing out the meaning of instructions and problems) and association (the process by which an association between a behaviour and a stimulus is learnt; the assumption that ideas and experiences reinforce one another and can be linked to enhance the learning process), instead of the usual lower order thinking skill of recall that results from rote learning (Boaden et al 1999). Students can achieve this learning through modes such as placements in community institutions and resources, observing doctors and members of the health team, and data collection and dissemination (reports, etc). Classroom and clinical-based methods such as lectures, and observation of experts can also aid the teaching-learning process.

Eraut's (1994) second type of professional knowledge is personal knowledge and the interpretation of experience. This category refers to knowledge that the student gains passively from experiences that are not openly related to learning, particularly in situations where the concentration is to try and do things. Such learning experiences must be planned so that teachers and students can employ teaching and learning strategies and resources that shift the responsibility of searching and using information to the learner. For example, such learning steps can begin with motivating students to analyse their life-experiences, followed by arrangements that provide students the chance for discovery and reflection, and later, introducing students to theories and to abstract and general ideas. Eventually, students are provided opportunities to develop skills in developing plans, action planning and implementation of plans. Community health educators must work out or adapt the teaching/learning strategies and resources that will suit such student-oriented learning processes, such as one-to-one teaching in the community that includes problem-solving, self-assessment and similar teaching and learning strategies.

Erauts's (1994) third category of professional knowledge is process knowledge, which makes great use of propositional (or content) knowledge and is, according to Eraut, at the centre of professional practice. Process knowledge refers to knowing how to do things. Here, the student acquires and orders information, develops skilled behaviour (complex sequence of routinised actions), uses deliberative processes (e.g. planning, evaluating, analysing and decision making) gives information (e.g. communicates appropriately) and monitors him/herself (audit on activities in his or her practice). As has been mentioned earlier, there is increasing need to strengthen and expand the preparation of health professionals for roles in PHC/Community Health, as evidence from the relevant literature indicates. For example, a global study (Hirschfeld et al 1997) to examine the strengthening of nursing and midwifery services showed that globally there is agreement that nurses and midwives should obtain more community health education than is now available.

In addition, the study identified not only needs for better preparation in PHC, but also needs for more skills in PHC in the community and in nurse clinics, and in work in different sectors of health care systems. Despite the problems the objectives approach to curriculum planning pose, the approach, as already mentioned, can be valuable especially where some kind of clear goals as a prerequisite for being a rational activity is required, such as in planning the teaching of important tasks in clinical settings like the health centre where, for example, patients from PHC villages are referred. In such community clinical settings, the students should be assisted to acquire basic skills (acceptable "core"), which, as we indicated earlier, translates to a level of achievement, their understanding and ability in crucial areas of knowledge and skills that the student can use in adult and working-life. These skills should be broad-based and transferable, rather than specific and job-restricted, and should include that range known as social and life skills.

Boaden et al (1999) describe another useful model that demonstrates how learning in community can be achieved in the planning of student and faculty activities in the community through the use of the logical, psychological, social and scientific principles and the concepts and principles of education, learning and PHC/ community health we outlined in chapters of Part One. This model demonstrates the usefulness of both the descriptive and prescriptive curriculum models, including the curriculum process model whose application, as Goodson et al (1975) suggest, requires teachers to describe the type of encounter which best characterises the new procedure through cooperative learning. This is the fourth stage of Boaden et al's model (also discussed in detail in Part One, Chapter 5, and in the following section).

The model (Boaden et al 1999) consists of four educational stages for learning clinical skills in the community. In the first stage (exploration) the student starts his/her experience of the community as a setting for clinical work. For instance, the student gets used to the new environment, observes and follows a senior doctor and mentor; he or she conducts some interviews, and uses some diagnostic tools. The student then progresses to the second and third educational stages in the development of clinical skills in the community (skill development and increasing independence in learning, respectively).

At the second stage the student is, for example, exposed more widely to the community and the practice environment; he or she takes more history and engages in clinical procedures under supervision, and discusses management plans. At the third stage the student, for example, performs clinical skills in a more reasonable period with minimal supervision, improves presentations and case writing skills, draws up a differential diagnosis, takes part in clinical audit, and is increasingly aware of community networks. At the fourth stage of development of clinical learning (co-operative learning) the student is capable of carrying out certain critical actions such as unsupervised practice, using effective communications skills, learning with others, using community and referral procedures appropriately, and involving members of the team appropriately.

During 1998 - 2000, an international team of five researchers described nine innovative health profession education programmes as selected by The Network: Community Partnerships for Health through Innovative Education. Based upon an analysis of the cases, Richards (2001) presents seven "lessons learned" as well as a discussion of programme development, institutionalisation of reform and long-term implications for health professions education. Two of the lessons learned have particular relevance for the design of student activities in the community. One is that student activities are determined based upon sensitivity to locale. While it is recognised that there is a unifying body of knowledge and an underlying set of skills, competencies and proclivities needed by all graduates, the context of practice is an overwhelming factor.

Teachers and their students need to ask: what are the pressing health needs of the population who will become the graduates' patients? What do "incidence and prevalence" mean in the place(s) where the graduates will practise? If infant mortality is high, why is it high? How do people access care? What technology is available at the local clinic? What are the implications of these questions for curriculum development and student learning? All the examples require students to rotate through community-based practice sites that range from rural village assignments to neighbourhood-based primary care clinic system, to a mobile health-care van that travels the back roads of localities. To prepare students to work under variable conditions, first and foremost, the curriculum is planned to stress patient examination skills and problem-solving methods. Core competencies for practitioners include using simple equipment such as the stethoscope, combined with a communication style that elicits a complete patient profile, and the ability to perform a detailed physical examination. Included in each programme are early contact with patients and most of the programmes stress history-taking and patient instruction at the beginning of the programme. Additionally, many programmes use Problem- Based Learning (PBL) (see Part 1, Chapter 3) to prepare students to proceed from most common to least common diagnoses.

The other important lesson learned is that teachers and students work collaboratively with other health professions. Most programmes in this study maintain an interdisciplinary approach to teaching primary health care. Some programmes even have all health professions students participate in the same foundation courses. Depending on the programme, this may or may not include PBL tutorials. Faculty in one institution, for instance, has developed a Rural Track, an interdisciplinary curriculum using the cohort approach. Twenty-five per cent of the students choose this option. Students select a rural community to learn in and the cohort stays together for the remaining two years of their education. Rural Track courses are team-taught by faculty from nursing, medicine and public as well as allied health. Teachers and students are not differentiated by discipline. In another institution students start their education with an intensive interdisciplinary PBL tutorial. Interdisciplinary opportunities are included throughout the curriculum. Towards the end of their course of study, students rotate through the Student Training Ward, an eight-bed in-patient orthopaedic unit. Most patients are elderly and present with orthopaedic problems complicated by underlying medical conditions and social care needs. Students from medicine, nursing, physiotherapy and occupational therapy operate as a team and assume full charge of the ward under the supervision of an orthopaedic surgeon, a resident and a nurse in charge. The students conduct daily rounds and provide medical treatment, nursing care, occupational therapy and physiotherapy.

However, as Boaden et al (1999, p.53) say "much current innovation (in community-based medical education that aims to provide, direct supervised experience of the current specialty in the setting where it is normally practised) is driven by relatively modest objectives and arises within the well-established professional framework which adopts a relatively narrow primary care model (Part One, Chapter 1) of community-based health care. This rather conservative approach no doubt reflects the difficulties in establishing change, both within the institutions of medical education and across the structures of health care with their long-standing established patterns of professional dominance and relatively poor in-agency and inter-professional cooperation".

Furthermore, as the foregoing discussion shows, many community health institutions engaged in education that promotes cooperative and collaborative learning in the community, such as interdisciplinary learning, implemented new educational approaches without much attention to the possible need for modification of existing management strategies and structures. In other instances, alternative semi-autonomous organisational arrangements were set up by the established schools (Kahssay 1998). Although many educational institutions for health professionals have, as we have seen, undoubtedly tried to improve this situation by adopting existing relevant organisational arrangements or devising new ones, on the basis of the differing ideas on education, the result has still been a proliferation of many different and sometimes conflicting managerial arrangements in educational institutions and clinical settings (ibid), which arguably include managerial and educational arrangements for cooperative and collaborative learning.

These lessons suggest not only a growing interest in cooperative and collaborative learning in community health education, but also a need for community health educators to understand the methods of the cooperative and collaborative modes of learning in the community and how to use them in such education most effectively. The following sections deal with these issues.

**Cooperative and Collaborative Learning in Community Health Education**

The commonality between cooperative and collaborative learning is that they both incorporate group work, but collaboration entails the whole process of learning, not just cooperation (Brufee 1995). Collaborative learning may encompass modes like students teaching the teacher, students teaching one another, and of course the teacher teaches the students, too. More significantly, it signifies that students are responsible for one another's learning as well as their own and that reaching the goal implies that students have assisted one another to understand and learn (ibid). Contrarily, the process of cooperative learning is designed to enhance the attainment of a particular goal or product by people working together in groups, and most of what is going on in the class is still controlled by the teacher, even if the students are working in groups (ibid). On the other hand, collaborative learning is aimed at getting the students to take almost full responsibility for working together, changing and evolving together, and of course building knowledge together.

Brufee (1995) further simplifies the definitions of cooperative and collaborative learning by differentiating between foundational knowledge and non-foundational knowledge and makes the relationship between these two types of knowledge to collaborative and cooperative learning. Brufee associates non-foundational knowledge with the collaborative learning approach. Non-foundational knowledge can be understood as knowledge which is derived through reasoning; questioning, discussion and negotiation of beliefs (see Process curriculum model, Chapter 3). In contrast, foundational knowledge (or propositional knowledge as referred to by Eraut above), is understood as the basic knowledge (or foundation courses) - e.g. anatomy, physiology, biochemistry, etc (see Subject-centred curriculum model, Part One, Chapter 3). According to Brufee (1995), this is best learnt through cooperative learning structures.

Both types of knowledge and the cooperative and collaborative modes of learning linked to them are indicated in the descriptions of the frameworks on learning in the community and the exemplars from the study on innovative professional health education outlined above. For example, Eraut's (1994) suggestion that students should use propositional knowledge through the higher order thinking skills of replication, application, interpretation and association corresponds with structuring activities for transiting from cooperative to collaborative learning, which Table 38 demonstrates. Also, as we can see, Boaden et al (1999) have outlined in their description student actions in cooperative learning as a final step in student learning in the community.

Thus, what is required of community health educators functioning in the community setting is to help effect changes that will enhance such attempts in applying cooperative and collaborative learning techniques in the community. To do this they must firstly strive for a clear understanding of the cooperative and collaborative learning modes, as well as the learning frameworks that correspond with them, such as interdisciplinary learning. As we have already seen, not only do many pedagogical and curricular approaches contribute to the community of learning idea, the term among other things, is used in a rather loose way and there does not appear to have been much open conceptualisation. We have therefore in this book used the collaborative and cooperative modes of learning as the chief means through which the educational aspects of building a community of learning can be achieved, and have tried in chapters and sections of the book to outline the characteristics of these learning modes, the methods they use and how they can be applied most effectively in community health education. This helps to normalise the use of these two learning concepts in describing learning activities in the community so that the community health educator can make comparisons, and to make uniform the terms used.

It is, therefore, necessary for community health educators to develop not only understanding of the cooperative and learning modes, but also the skills needed for using the modes in community health settings. Table 38 shows how teacher and student activities can be structured to convert from cooperative learning to collaborative learning. The table can be a useful resource for teachers and their students who wish to learn the methods of cooperative and collaborative learning and how they can form activities to change from cooperative to collaborative learning. Chapter 11 discusses aspects of an online cooperative project (Dooly 2008) that can eventually be used as a fully collaborative learning project in community health and Table 38 can therefore serve as a useful introduction to that discussion. As we indicated earlier, in order to meet the requirements of 'a renewed primary health care system' professionals will be required to collaborate to develop comprehensive plans of care. This will require professionals to take the time to get to know the skills that different professional groups bring to the primary health care setting. Primary health care teams will be challenged, among other things, to incorporate differing frames through which to develop an understanding of, and responsiveness to, the changing needs of the communities they serve. As already mentioned, one of the five areas for action the WHO (1987) has identified for a renewed PHC is development of individual personal skills.

Table 38: Structuring Activities for Transiting from Cooperative to Collaborative Learning

| | | General Definitions | | | Specific Instructional Elements | |
|---|---|---|---|---|---|---|
| | **Group: processes & management** | **Individual self-direction of Learning** | **Topic Selection** | **Learning Processes** | **Identification of Resources** | **Learning Outcomes** |
| **Level 1** (Structuring for lowest level SDL & Col; most structured level of scaffolding | Teacher will group according to Jigsaw method, determine roles and tasks for each group member, direct all instructional activities,monitor the group, etc. Students' roles are primarily to follow directions and participate in the group activities. | Teachers direct all individual learning activities, and students'are expected to follow directions. Progress and individual contributions are monitored by the teacher. Teachers help students to stay on-task, to try harder, and to contribute more. | Teacher assigns topics for expert and home groups in the Jigsaw setting. | describing what the students are to "hand in". Teacher communicates expectation for what the students should deliver, and can show model answers and outcomes | The list of resources is fixed by the teacher.Students engage with the same materials and resources with minimal variation. | The list of resources is fixed by the teacher. Students engage with the same materials and resources with minimal variation. |
| **Level 2** | Teacher sets guidelines for group formation and division of labour, students form their own groups accordingly. | Students can identify or reflect on their own learning and identify gaps, and how they are contributing to group activities | Teacher presents a limited list of possible topics/questions/problems. Students select from the list, or perhaps vote on the topic. | Students will decide what the final deliverable will be, but based on general guidelines from the teacher. | A starter list of resources is given, but students are encouraged to find their own, as well. The teacher might suggest search strategies or how to "filter" information. | The teacher lays out the various communication or production requirements, but students will agree among themselves who will be responsible for what. Students can explain why the various duties were allocated the way they were. |

| | | | | | | |
|---|---|---|---|---|---|---|
| | After establishing the basics students decide for themselves task management, task allocation, consulting with the teacher when problems arise. The teacher closely monitors the groups' processes and progress, but refrains from "hand-holding". | Teachers and peer leaders to play key roles to help each student to meet their learning needs, and to encourage sharing, communication and participation. | Teacher might facilitate a brainstorming activity to generate lists of possible topics/questions | The teacher also tries to trigger ideas, and/or to encourage creativity or unique responses. Students might make their choices based on a limited set of options given by the teacher. | | |
| **Level 3** (Structuring for highest level of SDL & Col; least structured level of scaffolding) | Groups are expected to form on their own, manage their own progress, divide up tasks, establish milestones, monitor progress, and troubleshoot problems. Teachers act as stimulators, coaches, facilitators and consultants, not as managers. | Students identify their own strengths and weaknesses and learning gaps for the task, and devise strategies to bridge the gaps and monitor learning progress. Teachers act as facilitators and consultants, not as managers. | Students have a free choice of topics/questions/problems according to their own decision-making process (voting, consensus, etc.). | Students set their own agenda for what they want to achieve or deliver, but will seek experts' help when necessary. The teacher consults and encourages, but refrains from showing "model answers or projects". | Students are to locate, select, and filter resources relevant to the learning task. | The final presentation and communication are organised, allocated and managed by the team. Both team and individual elements are highly productive and functional. |

Source: Learning Sciences and Technologies Academic Group, NIE (2010)

The approach shown in Table 38 is required for applying cooperative and collaborative methods in the community. Generally, learning methods used in the community can be categorized as (Boaden et al 1999): (1) methods and techniques suited to classroom-based activities such as the lecture, case discussion and small group work and (2) techniques and methods whose main aim is to use experience as a basis for learning and include clinical activities and those grounded in field work within the wider community. Such learning methods and techniques can also be used in cooperative and collaborative learning in the community. This is because cooperative and collaborative learning techniques, as can be seen from previous discussions, revolve around the use of small groups learning activities, as many of the other teaching techniques do. They can be used with almost any other educational strategy. The cooperative and collaborative learning techniques described here will help community health educators and students make the best use of small-group activities. Utilisation of the small-group in backgrounds like the clinics as a learning setting is perhaps the best example here. As already mentioned, the educational justification of this strategy is two-fold. First, students can be gently, but firmly, imbued with the attitude that it is desirable and enjoyable to learn and work harmoniously in groups with other pupils. Second, the small-group strategy has the advantage of creating possibilities for students to learn the values and skills of inter-working with other members of the multidisciplinary health team.

To apply cooperative and collaborative learning methods and techniques in the community, the teacher must focus on communities, homes, schools, industries, hospitals, and other institutions, as the primary settings for learning, not the lecture or large discussion groups. The role of the learner and the teacher in the community is generalised and interdependent within the health sector and health-related sectors; the concerns of both student and teacher are the prevailing health problems and needs of the community, the approach to their practice is primary health care which demands community/family/patient participation in care, identification and follow-up of vulnerable groups, and the health team approach.

The student and teacher are engaged in problem-solving activities, involving community/group/family/individual needs and resources, and assessing interventions through community/group/family/individual. The objectives of practice concentrate on primary prevention and therapeutic care aimed at improving patient, family, and community health, and self-care. All these happen within a health delivery system that is based on the premise of primary health care for all, involving other sectors that influence health, and using the health team approach. Also, the evaluation of health care practice focuses on percentage of coverage of population, service utilisation rates by high-risk groups, and the rates of change in health status of high-risk groups/communities.

Much of this may be included in the programmes described above. It is however useful to clearly specify these requirements of the PHC approach which, as we have seen in Part One, Chapter 1, constitutes the basis for studying and delivering community health in especially developing countries. For as Boaden et al (1999) point out present innovations in community- based education are pushed to a degree by mediocre objectives that come from the strong professional body which uses a relatively limited primary care model (Part One, Chapter 1). This constraints change both in health educational institutions and wider health care systems. Earlier in the discussion, we put forward strong arguments in favour of using the cooperative and collaborative modes of learning in the community. As discussed, these approaches to learning in the community can engage students in many activities to form the social interactions needed to establish and build community of learning in community health. They can create community in the absence of important faculty involvement. Also, by using these learning frameworks faculty can have a great positive impact on shaping, contributing to, and extending the learning environment of students in the community. The ICT-supported collaborative learning concept is important for another reason. It gets students to build knowledge together which, as already indicated, enhances the student's education in community health where after his/her education they will have to deal with the realities that predispose community health. Furthermore, ICT-supported cooperative and collaborative teaching and learning reflect the push to preparing students in community health to be responsible citizens in an increasingly technologically advanced world.

Network-based learning is an excellent way to plan tasks that incorporate strategies for providing students with opportunities to learn higher order thinking skills in groups within the cooperative and collaborative learning modes either synchronously or asynchronously. The following section considers how teachers and their students can use synchronous and asynchronous learning methods in combination with ICT-supported cooperative and collaborative learning in community health education.

## Synchronous and Asynchronous Learning Facilitation and Delivery in the Community

As discussed, the best method for exchanging information, communication and opinions as well as the choice of ICT tool for doing this will depend on many contextual factors, such as the objectives of the overall project, age of students, the group personality and local constraints. As in applying cooperative and collaborative learning in the community, teachers and students can also use traditional learning methods and techniques in synchronous and asynchronous learning in the community. The asynchronous approach, for example, combines self-study with asynchronous interactions to promote learning, and it can be used to facilitate learning not only in traditional on-campus education, but also in distance and continuing education which can be conducted in the community. However, in the community the teacher and student roles, student and teacher activities, as well as the objectives of student practice assume different characteristics from those undertaken in traditional educational settings. Gretchen et al (2011) explore and compare the differences between asynchronous and synchronous learning facilitation strategies, facilitators and learner roles, and delivery within a synchronous and asynchronous learning environment, which the following section presents with information from the community health education literature.

**Facilitation Strategies**

Teaching strategies for synchronous and asynchronous learning environments vary because the learning environment depends on differences of time and place. Facilitators of synchronous learning provide an experience similar to the traditional learning environment (Gretchen et al 2011). Synchronous instructors are proactively interacting with students during class time. The asynchronous learning environment is similar to the online modality or distance education courses (ibid).

## Synchronous

**Facilitation Strategies**

- Provide visuals through webcasts or webinars. This allows the learners to follow you through your presentation.
- Using PowerPoint, blackboard or whiteboards can reinforce performance objectives visually.
- Activate an auditory element through podcast or webcast. The inflection in your voice will help to reinforce learning for auditory learners.
- Chat capabilities allow students to brainstorm, collaborate or ask questions with verbally interrupting the presentation and are essential for multi-tasking.
- Save teleconferences or webinars, so that students can refer back to them at a later date.

## Asynchronous

**Facilitation Strategies**

- Incorporate activities that empower student collaboration outside of forum discussion.
- Provide students with a timeline or calendar that promotes proactive participation in discussion forums.
- Facilitate by using your online personality. Use emoticons to showcase your personality. Be cognisant of being too "wordy" or not providing enough explanations for assignments.
- Promote forum discussions by using open-ended questioning methods.
- Provide audio and visual links to meet the needs of different learning styles.

**Roles of Facilitator and Learner**

When deciding to enrol in an adult education course, choosing an online forum compared to a face-to-face modality is only part of the decision. Whether you are the instructor or student deciding on asynchronous or a synchronous modality will change the form of communication and expectations during the course. The following shows differences in the roles that the facilitator, instructor or student play in synchronous and asynchronous modalities.

## Synchronous

**Facilitator**

- Manage late arrivals to class meetings
- Must be comfortable in front of camera or microphone. Prepared for any technological issues that may arise. Prepared with different strategies to keep the students involved and participating in discussions.
- Facilitator or instructor must be able to multi-task while encouraging the students to actively participate, pose questions that will keep the students involved. Preparing a series of questions will help the instructor to anticipate questions and responses immediately.
- Facilitator can use different tools to keep the students involved, engaged and participating in the course. Present material for a period of time then have a period of time for the students to participate by asking questions, adding experience or point of view to the discussion.

## Asynchronous

**Facilitator**

- Tracks participation and attendance
- Can prepare for entire course prior to the beginning. Complete with discussion questions, assignments and presentations. Including presentations in this forum allows the students to create presentations where they can utilise other web tools.
- Must answer promptly; however, there is a pause in time to prepare a thoughtful response. Only have to respond to one question or response at a time. Can ask follow up questions for further engagement of the students.
- Can see when the students are falling behind or not understanding the information presented. In this modality, the instructor can offer other tools to help the student comprehend the information.

## Synchronous

**Learner**

- Schedules time to attend live meetings.
- Focuses on discussions and live meetings. Avoid outside distractions and be able to actively participate.
- Seeks clarification on misunderstandings and misinterpretations and receive immediate feedback
- Has a real-time interaction with other students and instructor.

## Asynchronous

**Learner**

- Posts assignments, etc, when convenient during class each week.
  Is self-motivated to complete assignments and posts. No set time to be on computer
- Can ask questions of other students or instructor and receive clarification

any time of the day.

- Participates 24/7. Limits are set by learner staying organised and involved in the course of discussion and participation.

**Asynchronous Delivery**

As we have seen, a blog is a blend of the term Web log. As most blogs are interactive providing commentary or news on a particular subject or interest, it is the type of technology that lends itself to an educational environment, particularly adult education. It allows the educator to be more creative in preparing the class and permits the students to link with one another and the instructor in a collaborative and knowledge sharing environment.

The choice of a blog is appropriate for the adult learner in that it allows the student to attend and participate in class discussions and topics within a flexible time frame. Asynchronous delivery medium works well with adult learners in that it gives them time to reflect before entering into a discussion as well rewrite agreements or rebuttals on any type of subject matter. The answer is generally thought out to a greater extent than in a synchronous medium.

Blogs as a mode of delivery could be applied to a current adult education teaching environment as blogs are public and allow for interaction and active collaboration of ideas and disciplines; these are easily transferred to diverse groups of learners. Finding blogs that are relevant to the students are relatively easy. Blog posting brings together many different articles through links as well as many points of view on a particular subject from around the web (ibid).

A synchronous medium such as a Power Point presentation can also get the instruction across and has been used in both classrooms and training for quite some time. The Power Point presentation can engage learners on a particular subject but does not allow collaboration other than inducing discussion for later attention (ibid).

The application of especially blogs as a method of delivering education in community health is important as many of the students in community health schools may be adults who, as the theory of adult learning assumes, have a need to be self-directed and to know why they are learning something; they are motivated to learn by intrinsic as well as extrinsic factors; they enter into a learning experience with a problem-centred approach to learning, and adults bring more work-related experiences into the learning environment (ibid).

However, the delivery of blogs, like any other ICT applications in education, must consider the applicability of ICTs in community health education settings. As Trucano (2005) also suggests, it is clear that it is the application of various ICTs that are the most important determinants of the effectiveness of such tools in education. While ICT can enhance interactions among many actors in teaching and learning processes, the role played by ICT in the process of collaboration, however, is not always supportive of learning. This is because ICT can at times just be a communication channel that is neutral to learning (Sing et al 2001).

Sing et al (2001) contrast ICT as communication channel with ICT for collaborative meaning making, and highlight that not all utility supports collaborative learning. ICT as communication channel refers to the use of ICT mainly for enabling communication. There are learning situations where ICT is used as a communication channel for members within a group to interact with one another. Such communication can take place either in class to complement face-to-face interaction, or outside class as an extension or replacement of face-to-face interaction (with the latter being more predominant). In such situations, the focus really is to enable talk among students and sometimes with the teacher, and less emphasis is placed on whether the talk leads to learning. Likewise, ICT for collaborative meaning making can occur within class or outside class. However, the similarity ends there. Rather than be concerned with how ICT enables talk among students, what matters is how features of ICTs influence the course of collaboration. In other words, how students use ICTs in group settings. Thus, taken in this light, students can be using ICT even in a face-to-face setting so long as the interaction works towards collaborative meaning making. This makes cooperative/collaborative learning systems fundamentally social technologies that mediate and encourage actions by collaborators to achieve learning.

Comparisons of synchronous and asynchronous learning environments (Hayes 2012) found that the most beneficial learning environments is a blended course with both synchronous and asynchronous instruction for online learning environments to ensure the needs of all learning styles, as well as enhance students' learning capabilities. There are advantages and disadvantages to synchronous and asynchronous learning environments that community health educators should be aware of. Table 39 presents advantages and disadvantages of synchronous and asynchronous learning.

**Table 39: Advantages and disadvantages of synchronous and asynchronous learning**

| **Advantages**<br>***Synchronous learning*** | **Disadvantages**<br>***Synchronous learning*** |
|---|---|
| • Widely offered by schools in online education<br>• Cost effective.<br>• Permits immediate feedback and detailed collaboration both with instructors and fellow students.<br>• Physical barriers of distance are eliminated.<br>• Global and accessible for all learners.<br>• Flexibility<br>• Enhances self-esteem, confidence, and work performance<br>• Technologies such as email, classroom discussion forum, individual forums, and team forums facilitate interactions between learners and the instructor. | • Learners who lack proficient or basic computer skills may struggle or drop the class.<br>• Learners who lack self-confidence, guidance, self-teaching skills and lack of motivation.<br>• Different time zones which may affect scheduling and participation issues.<br>• Sense of being disconnected from the group that students may potentially develop.<br>• Due to learners feeling of disconnect learner may lack motivation.<br>• Learners see the course as an obstacle and develop an adversarial relationship with the instructor.<br>• Learners who lack communication or social skills may not succeed in the class. |

| **Advantages**<br>*Asynchronous learning* | **Disadvantages**<br>*Asynchronous learning* |
|---|---|
| • Overwhelmingly positive impact on the overarching learning objectives for most courses.<br>• All comments from the students and the instructor are saved throughout the class and organised by discussion and date.<br>• Generally beneficial for learners who take poor notes or forced to attend extremely overcrowded traditional face-to-face classrooms.<br>• Self-motivated learners.<br>• Learners in control of their learning. | • Sense of being disconnected from the group that students may potentially develop.<br>• Due to learners feeling of being disconnected learner may lack motivation.<br>• Learners may see the course as an obstacle and develop an adversarial relationship with the instructor. |

Table 35 also provides pointers that community health educators can consider in applying the cooperative and collaborative learning modes, as well as other pedagogical and curricular approaches that can enhance a community of learning in community health education.

**Summary**

This chapter discussed features of effective pedagogical, curricular and co-curricular design that incorporate the elements of building a community of learning, offering examples and conceptual interpretations based on training programmes and frameworks drawn from the education, management and community health literature. It looked at the curriculum design process and provided a multiple curricular approach that agrees with building a community of learning in community. It discussed the designing of student and faculty pedagogical and curricular activities in the community, with particular reference to the cooperative and collaborative learning modes, as well as synchronous and asynchronous learning through which students can experience network learning within the cooperative and collaborative learning techniques. These approaches to learning serve as the main means of accomplishing the educational aims of the broader concept of a community of learning.

The following chapter looks at how collaborative and cooperative learning can be further enhanced by setting up ICT-supported collaborative and cooperative learning projects in community health. As will be seen, the chapter provides guidelines on how community health educators can use various ICTs to achieve cooperative and collaborative learning goals in the community.

# 11

## *Designing Online Cooperative and Collaborative Learning Projects in Community Health*

In Part One, Chapter 4, we briefly explained a working definition of cooperative and collaborative learning and why it is important. A brief overview of how the premise of constructivism provides an important axis for collaborative and cooperative work and how this type of approach easily fits with online learning is given. Dooly (2008) has described an online cooperative project that can eventually be used as a fully collaborative learning project. This chapter discusses aspects of the project design with reference to building a community of learning in community health, giving examples and theoretical explanations from the education and community health relevant literature, as well as the writer's experience in the area. This chapter outlines the significance of online collaborative and cooperative projects, providing tips on how to select a project partner and come up with a good project idea. This is followed by steps to use during the planning stage. In the implementation stage, how to set up groups and manage the group work are described. Finally, a few useful guidelines on finishing the project are outlined. As Dooly (2008) suggests, it may be difficult for teachers in ideal community health contexts to implement a full collaborative learning process in which students are completely autonomous and all the team members negotiate and decide the tasks or activities on their own. However, it can be a goal to strive for in community health. This chapter helps those who wish to achieve such a goal.

### The importance of online collaborative and cooperative learning projects in community health education

As we have already seen in Part One, Chapter 4, students can perform at higher intellectual levels in collaborative situations than when working individually. Also, group diversity can contribute positively to the learning process. There are several reasons for this: (1) students are faced with various interpretations, explanations or answers about what they are studying and this forces them to review their own viewpoints. Including network-based learning into the process of collaborative learning can therefore be very beneficial in terms of knowledge and experience because students will be working with a diverse student group and this interaction may bring them to re-formulate some of their ideas (2) network-based collaboration may provide opportunities for more equality in group work than actual face-to-face group work, since in the latter approach group "decision-making" is often contingent upon which student has the loudest voice or who has the most confidence in the target language. ICT tools (for example, discussion boards or web logs) can be so useful in the learning process because students who might be shy at voicing their opinion face-to-face now have the opportunity to express themselves and can take their time and think out carefully exactly what they wish to say (3) collaborative teaching reflects the push to preparing our students to be responsible citizens in an increasingly technologically advanced society (Dooly 2008).

However, it is not just a question of getting our students to sit down in front of a computer and, for example, begin chatting with a school partner in another country or asking them to find information about a country the teacher has arbitrarily chosen. The projects and activities that teachers ask the students to take part in, or activities the students choose themselves, should reflect the current and future needs of the learner. Lamberti (2012), who allowed his students to use computers in class for activities such as writing or building websites, describes an incident in which he asked his students to open only the software he required them to use while they worked. Within five minutes of giving the instructions, most of the students were surfing the Internet while finishing the task he had given them. When questioned on their behaviour, the students justified it by saying they were multitasking: simultaneously writing, texting, reading websites, refreshing Facebook, listening to music, and watching TV online. This they explained made them 'roll'. Lamberti (2012) discovered that his students disliked conversing face-to-face and that their only news came from Facebook. Learners must learn to control technology and not let technology control them.

Moreover, students must be made aware that advances and changes in technology can and should be embraced as new possibilities. This is because the students in today's classrooms will be future job-seekers and that means learning to use not only the technological tools available today, but also technology tools they will use in their work in the future. One of these possibilities is using ICT tools as a means to effectively organising their work, in particular, working in a distanced team. The need for future workers in community health to be able to adapt to these type of work environments cannot be overemphasised. By stressing teamwork through ICT tools, the students will learn to think creatively, to solve problems, and to make decisions as a team. Additionally, they will be in control of technology and not slaves to it. Teachers must assist their students to learn to interact positively with people who are different from themselves and who may not think the same as they do. Whether it is through collaborative or cooperative learning, getting students to learn to work together in the classroom and with other students in another part of the world is crucial. Through online collaboration students may come to see the significance of taking responsibility for their own learning and feel empowered to do so while learning to respect the opinions and work of their online partners (Dooly 2008). Let us now look at the steps that community health teachers can follow to effectively implement cooperative and collaborative learning in the community.

**Finding a project idea and a project partner**

It does hold true that many ideas occur at moments when one least expects them, like while one is in a classroom, having a coffee break in the teachers' lounge, watching a film and so forth. However, the issues of getting a project idea can be dealt with in participatory processes of curriculum development (e.g. Tenn et al 1994). Brainstorming in such a process is a good way of coming up with ideas, mainly because the multidisciplinary team members know the general area of community health that they want to work in.

The multidisciplinary team can find a project idea by (1) having a look at the standard criteria in the project area. This can be at school, central or community level. This is to see the benchmarks expected at your students' level that can provide inspiration for the project design (2) finding out about the interests of your students or aspects of their daily life and trying to match these interests to the project design (3) tying the project to an event going on in the school or partner school or the local community.

It is best for teachers, students and their community collaborators to look for project ideas within parameters that they are familiar with in the community, making sure they have some knowledge of the topic themselves. They should look for inspiration around the community. They could build on or expand a previous project, go to local conferences for new ideas, look at events at their school or community that inspire them or go online to do some research about other projects. For example, these projects ideas (CQ University 2011) are reported on the Internet as part of a study to investigate the relationships between formal and informal education, community engagement and health:

- Health promotion and community engagement research projects that focus on changing individual, organisational and community health behaviour.
- Health promotion and community engagement research projects that focus on producing a health outcome at an individual, organisational and community level.
- Community-based education research projects that focus on producing a health outcome at an individual, organisational and community level.
- Research projects, including historical analyses that contribute to the understanding of the relationships between health, organisational and community engagement and education.
- Research projects that focus on the influence of cultural factors within communities and organisations on the learning and development of relationships between health sectors and staff to inform education.

- Learning and teaching research projects that inform teaching into health related programmes through building community and engagement amongst students.

Teachers, students and their community collaborators can also draw project ideas by focusing on the factors that affect community health and the tools of community health practice: epidemiology (the study of the distribution and determinants of diseases and injuries in human populations - data that are recorded as number of cases or as rates (number per 1,000 or 100,000); community organising (bringing people together to combat shared problems and increase their say about decisions that affect their lives, a developmental approach that is well emphasised in many chapters of this book); and health promotion (which involves health education and disease prevention programming, a process by which various interventions are planned, implemented, and evaluated for the purpose of improving or maintaining the health of a community or population (Green et al 2002).

As already mentioned, finding a partner can also happen in participatory processes of curriculum development. A partner in such a process may already know what he or she wants to do and is looking for a partner to "fit" the project profile. Or perhaps the potential partners already know each other and are simply interested in carrying out an online project but are not certain at this point about the outline of the project. As already mentioned, most community health schools have developed community-oriented experiences for students located in clinical practice settings in local communities, such as health centres and clinics. Their collaborators working in such practice settings that may be teachers from the schools, or other stakeholders in community agencies and organisations, as well as other community members, can ideally be useful project partners.

It is essential that the partners in the process take the time to get to know each other before beginning the project. This necessary social interaction can best take place through text chats, emails or voice chats, as well as face-to-face, informal and structured meetings. Part Two Chapter 1 outlines the five steps a faculty leader can take to harness the full potential of community and engaging community in designing the learning space, including understanding and appreciating different perspectives of team members.

Several websites are designed as portals for schools looking for Internet partners (Dooly 2008). Many of these portals provide examples and reports about successful projects and ideas which can inspire new projects. Dooly (2008) provides some examples: iEARN; NickNacks Telecollaborative Projects; Kidlink and Kidproj. For information about online science projects in a very large network, Dooly suggests seeing Global SchoolNet Foundation. Although, as she says, this site is mainly dedicated to science projects, it provides information about collaborative learning, examples of successful projects and access to possible partnerships.

An International Online Collaborative Health Project between the University of The Gambia Department of Nursing and the School of Nursing, Miami University, Ohio, demonstrates how a project idea and partner can be found (Sarr and Mason 2008). This assignment is a result of discussions on collaboration, as well as student and faculty exchanges between the two institutions that have been going on for several years. It is designed to provide opportunities for Bachelor of Science in Nursing (BSN) students of both universities to explore the contemporary and relevant public health issues affecting populations in both countries. The assignment is undertaken by the students in both countries as part of the community health courses in their study programmes. Thus, this collaboration provided a unique opportunity for selecting a project partner and an idea that appealed so well to international students and faculty.

**Preparatory or planning stage**

Again, this is a step that a participatory curriculum development committee can take with care. Teachers and students who are interested in implementing collaborative and cooperative learning should as a first step think of every stage in the group work in order to be able to provide support whenever required. This suggests bearing in mind the topics, activities or projects which are part of the regular curriculum and deciding which ones they would best adapt to the collaborative work they would like to implement. This also suggests thinking of how the students will be organised in groups during the collaboration. Teachers need to consider the following questions in order to organise their project into their curriculum:

1. Will the students do the activities during class time, outside of the class, or a bit of both? As discussed earlier in Part Two Chapter 2, it is necessary for teachers to discuss and plan with their project partners. Here, more details about how to build an efficient partnership with stakeholders are provided.
2. Have you included this work into the regular teaching plan?
3. What is the overall scope of the project (how long will it take, when will you start, when will you finish and so on?)
4. Have you discussed this with your project partner?

When deciding the scope of the project, teachers and their collaborators will need to consider the duration (e.g. a week to a month or most of the semester) and the breadth of the project (are you going to cover one topic or several integrated topics? (See the integrated curriculum model and other curriculum models in Part One, Chapter 3). The scope will help determine the number of stages, which must be planned. After teachers have a topic or idea, they should work backwards from there. They must go from the project idea to curriculum needs and desired output, etc. All these questions and points were considered during the planning of the International Online Collaborative Health Project.

**Inform students about what you are doing**

In Part Two, Chapter 8 on the learning space design steps, we highlighted the need for dialogue where everyone is heard and respected. Accordingly, teachers must make sure their students understand why they are asking them to participate in an online project and the underlying learning process. They should plan time into the beginning of the project to advise and explain to their students about the project. The need for making students comprehend the learning intentions is crucial. These must be explained to students in the best ways possible. Teachers should put learning goals in a wider context, such as "being able to communicate with others", for example. This agrees with the principles of the curriculum process model and other descriptive curriculum models described in Chapter 3. Teachers might get students to add their own ideas of what this means for them. This can be facilitated by providing students' examples of past projects, such as a PowerPoint presentation or a homepage.

**Teach the students to work collaboratively**

An important requirement in the participatory process of curriculum development is allotting enough time for serious reading of one another's work or getting comments from reviewers.

Time may also be needed to train students to work together. Teachers should consider activities from the point of view of individual tasks which, as a combined effort, make a whole. They should:

- make sure they have allocated time for training in group work
- decide with their project partner whether this will be done together as part of the project or if it is to be done before the project actually begins, and then set their timetable accordingly.

As students might not have worked in collaborative learning groups before, they may need training in group dynamics. Teachers should look for steps in preparing their students for group collaboration in useful resources like the Internet. This is important as it is suggested (Conlan et al 2003) that project-based learning might not always be the best learning method when dealing with many different cultures and backgrounds because problem-solving methods vary from culture to culture.

**Develop a Substitute Plan**

It is essential that each and every member or group in the participatory process of curriculum development should share with other members descriptions of the parts of the work they have been assigned. Likewise, it is necessary for group members to have the chance to view and to comment on any material that may have a bearing on the planning of their individual or group assignments. In this respect, teachers and their partners must always plan for contingencies. Including online collaborative learning projects into the curriculum requires a lot more strategic and logistic planning from the teacher than face-to-face plans. They must have alternative plans for "risk" situations (e.g. an individual in the group cannot or does not complete his/her task; or planned synchronous contact with the project partners fails due to technical difficulties, etc.). In the international online collaborative health project, such issues were dealt with through emails and telephone calls.

**Verify the Goals/Objectives**

Many of the learning theories we covered in Part One, Chapter 4, point to the requirement for teachers to identify trainees' needs and communicate how training programme content relates to fulfilling these needs, including the need to know why they are learning something. It is therefore important for teachers and their partners to double-check the goals (see for example, curriculum process model) to make sure that the work is relevant to the students' goals. This is because at first the novelty of online work will soon lose its appeal if the students do not see a reason for continuing to learn a topic. On the other hand, if the students are using the knowledge to build or discover new knowledge with their online companions, they will be motivated to continue and to take more and more risks with the topic of the lesson.

The goals/objectives of the international online collaborative assignment were to develop a proposal that will convince participants that contemporary and relevant health issues should be studied for better understanding and action. At the end of the assignment the students were expected to be able to:

1. Identify priority public health issues facing each country.

2. Outline relevant Health Policy Statements and Declarations which speak to priority health issues for each country such as:
   - The World Health Organisation's statement on "Health For All by the Year 2000"
   - "Healthy People 2010" (United States Document)

3. Compare and contrast the priority issues as they affect each country.

4. Decide on possible courses of action for tackling or addressing the priority issues in each country.

5. Write a report of their collaborative work and conclusions.

This information was disseminated among and within student groups in both countries (Sarr and Mason 2008). These were the goals/objectives that students considered important and strove to achieve:

**Be Ready to be Self-Critical**

Some people believe that geographic isolation of target groups, for example, makes participation impossible. However, it is possible to include most isolated groups with some creativity and time. The difficulty of integrating an online collaborative project into the goals and objectives of a course may be compounded by the fact that the teachers are working with one or more partner classes at a distance, such as health centres and clinics at the local level of PHC, or in a country abroad. Unavoidably, the class goals and/or objectives in each case will be different. There will be need to find an online project that is relevant for all the classes involved. This requires teachers collaborating with one another and with their community partners to negotiate the activities, the design of the project, the methods, the assessment, the timetable and deadlines, etc – even before the project begins. These way teachers can serve as role models to their students.

This was what happened in the international online collaborative health project between the school of nursing in The Gambia and that of Ohio University, USA (Sarr and Mason 2008). This was not an easy experience as it was the first time that both parties were engaged in such a project. Problems encountered included cross-cultural issues that emerged during the experience and the timing of interactions between partners in both countries. However, finding the online project and negotiating the design of the project was much easier, as it emerged as an educational need during collaborative talks between the two institutions.

**Pair tasks with abilities and skills**

As was shown in the planning of the international online collaborative health project, it is crucial to match activities and tasks with the students' skills and abilities. This may be more difficult if the partner classes have different levels, as can happen in health centres and clinics where there can be various learner groups, such as doctors, nurses, etc. However, this should not be a constraint for collaborative learning. This is because collaborative learning is about teaching each other, so different skills and abilities can be incorporated into the activities. It is important to scale the activities by allowing students to start with relatively easy tasks at the beginning and then gradually increase the difficulty level as students progress in their knowledge in both the topic and ability to collaborate. Besides, if the students are to teach each other, working out the timeline and activity plans carefully with your project partner is of paramount importance.

In the international online collaborative community health project (Sarr and Mason 2008) Gambian and Miami students collaborated via email to become acquainted and then compared and contrasted the types of health issues identified in each country. Each group worked in their designated groups in each country. There was a designated email leader in each group who coordinated the answers to questions and sent an email with these answers to the email leader in the other country, copied to the supervisor in each country.

The email leader had each student in the group provide an introduction to his/her fellow students in the other country that can be shared with the corresponding group. This helped everyone learn a little bit about one another and understand one another a little more. Questions that were used to help students introduce themselves focused on length of nursing service, what students like most about nursing, what they find most challenging about nursing, reasons for returning to school for their bachelor's degree, how they hope their degree will help them, where they work, live and their family (if they would like to), and their greatest concerns about the assignment.

**Check the Working Environment**

Community health teachers must be clear about their own and their students' working environment prior to entering a transnational collaboration. Therefore, they should ask themselves these questions:

- Did your students ever participate in collaborative work before?
- Did your students try to use ICT tools in their daily work?
- For how long did your students learn the foreign language you want to employ in the collaboration?

- What kind of ICT support is available (such as technicians, number of computers and time available)?
- Did the idea of the transnational collaborative project receive the support of the head teacher and your colleagues?

The lessons learnt from the international online collaborative health project (Sarr and Mason 2008) make these questions particularly important. While language was not a problem, as faculty and students in both countries spoke English as the official language, and the idea of the project received much support from the school authorities in both countries, students in The Gambia were less conversant with the use of ICT than their USA counterparts. Also, the needed ICT support was more lacking in The Gambia. At the beginning of the project, participants did not always have easy, similar, and regular access to the chosen technology. Difficulties with access resulted in frustration as well as an imbalance in the quality and quantity of contributions among participants. In addition, the software and hardware (Bulletin Board, etc) between partner countries were not always compatible and user-friendly. Consequently, the teachers and students resorted to using emails and telephone calls.

**Implement the project**

After planning the activity sequences or "project map" and after negotiating the management issues with your partner, teachers can now go on to involve their students in the initiation of the project. The project map or "workflow" is just a brief outline of the main steps, which will be used when implementing the project and it is written to help the teachers and partners to think about how to carry out the project.

The outline that follows focuses mainly on getting the students ready for collaborative work, especially in the case of students who are not used to these activities.

**Clarify how the groups will operate**

If the group is not used to these types of activities, the teacher must carefully explain how the groups will operate and clearly specify each group task, making sure that the group is aware of the goals/objectives of the task and that they understand all relevant concepts.

In our international online collaborative health project (Sarr and Mason 2008), students were provided opportunities to discuss priority health issues between the two countries by means of online collaboration. Students were encouraged to make comparisons between the two countries, comparing and contrasting findings between countries, writing a report of findings and proposing solutions, and presenting findings and proposed solutions. The work of the groups in each country was supervised by a senior faculty member in each country, who provided students with ICTs and methods to communicate in learning environments, the course syllabus and calendar that was used for information regarding the course schedule and assignments, as well as communicating as frequently as possible with the students and with one another through private email, telephone and face-to-face meetings individually and in class. As the course progressed, the supervisors reviewed and reorganised the learning strategies as suggested by Stoner (1999).

**Use various ways to set up the groups**

The teacher can set up the groups or allow the groups to decide their members themselves. Some teachers may choose to pre-select the groups according to skills or past performances. In the international online collaborative health project students were placed by the teachers in three groups (A, B & C) in each country and provided opportunities to discuss such issues by means of online collaboration.

**Consider group size**

Often having more than four members per group decreases the chance for collaborative work. It is therefore wise to keep numbers in mind as well when building the online partnerships. This rule applies also to when considering the amount of time available for the online collaboration, matching the time available with the size of the group. As already mentioned, timing of interactions in the international online community health project was difficult because of the different time zones in the two countries. For this and other practical reasons, the group size was limited to three-five members.

**Assist students to be autonomous**

Teachers may have to provide very exact instructions about the learning process, depending on the group autonomy. While this may not be collaborative learning, it may be necessary in the beginning to ensure that the students start well. Instructions to students should include:

- how they should get started
- the kind of participation anticipated from the learners
- the way in which the task will be concluded

As in the international online collaborative health project (Sarr and Mason 2008), these instructions are incorporated in a hand-out sheet that lists the main elements of the collaborative process to enable the students to refer to it during the process. Students who are conversant with collaborative work can discuss the work among themselves. Such negotiation can be facilitated by asking the students to draw up written contracts which outline the members' obligations to their group, incorporating deadlines.

**Avoid making changes to the groups**

Teachers should follow this rule, even when things are not going well with the group. In particular, teachers should resist students' demands to be re-assigned. This is because changing groups may break the dynamics of all the groups. Additionally, the members of this group will not learn the essential part of collaborative learning, which is to resolve problems and manage difficult situtations. Giving in to changes can also undermine the students' belief in the importance of collaboration.

## Make students comprehend the plan of action

Giving the students the autonomy to deciding their own tasks and assigning the roles will depend on their skills and capabilities. In situations where students are given such autonomy, they should decide on activities for getting to know their online partners. If the students are incapable of carrying out this activity themselves, then it may be conducted by the teacher. Enough time should be given to students to negotiate their tasks. It is suggested that there should be written commitment from each group.

Where the students are yet to achieve complete collaborative learning, or lack the language skills necessary to negotiate the tasks with their partners, it may be necessary to assign them various roles that will help them to work together to construct knowledge. For example, a student can be given the role of a group motivator who will encourage members of the group to participate in the activities.

## Students should not be expected to be outgoing and friendly on cue

Although the aim is to strive for collaborative learning, teachers should not expect even the most autonomous students to select their own online partner. This is because it is difficult for students to introduce themselves to students who may be stranger and then start to work with them immediately. The teacher should decide if it is best to assign directly the online partner or group. Such a decision should be made by the collaborating teachers before starting the project. Teachers should give the students time and activities to get to know each other before they have to begin working together. This is vital to the well being of the project. Different activities can be combined with a view to getting students to know one another and select their partners at the same time.

To facilitate success of the discussion in the international online collaborative community health project (Sarr and Mason 2008), clear and specific guidelines for the amount (and type) of interaction required were provided (Merron 1999). Accordingly, this approach was designed to provide a place for nurses from different sides of the world to discuss common health concerns/problems. The aim was to encourage interaction among students not simply to present information, but to make comparisons between the two countries, comparing and contrasting findings between countries. Every student was free to present their ideas regarding these health issues. Students were advised that they were not competing with each other during discussion and that part of the expectations for their participation was that they contributed to one another's learning. It was considered a place for students to ask questions and assist other students with their questions.

Questions for clarification were highly encouraged. The goal for each group was to learn as much about the health priorities of the other country as possible and to recognise the roles that nurses can play to advance the health of the people. Students were required to forward their contributions in a constructive manner by a stated date. All students are nursing colleagues, and all opinions deserve a fair hearing and respect. Students were also held to academic standards of writing style and the use of proper grammar, punctuation and spelling. To stay on top of the assignment students needed to check their emails frequently.

**Ensure students know their responsibilities and possible consequences of non-participation**

Teachers should communicate clearly to students that their work plan includes a plan for dealing with members of the group who do not fulfil their responsibilities. While the students are writing their own work plans, they should decide how they wish to deal with such members.

Because students may be overly zealous or afraid of retaliation, teachers can give them some reasonable suggestions on how to deal with such members.

**Get groups to give regular feedback on their progress**

Outlines, drafts, worksheets to fill out, newspaper articles, discussion board reports, group minutes, oral presentations, or many other methods, as the international online collaborative community health project demonstrates, can serve as the means by which the teacher is informed about the groups' progress and the students to learn or assimilate skills (presentations, article writing, etc.). The updates on student progress should be shared online. In addition, the collaborating teachers should ensure that they maintain open communication about progress and/or problems in each of the classes involved in the project.

**Final stage**

Closure follows the completion of the learning activities. An important aspect of closure is, needless to say, course assessment. The way to do this can be challenging because the teachers are assessing the collaborative learning process and not just the end product. Alternatively, teachers can involve the students in the process through modes such as group evaluation, peer evaluation and self-assessment. The teachers can ask their students to assess their group's work, for example; however, the students should give reasons for their evaluation, not only provide marks. A team report (written collaboratively) and/or an individual report can be ways teachers can do this. Various ICT formats can be included in the assessment process, such as e-portfolios, online voting systems, news articles, etc. In addition, teachers can also self-assess the project and ask students to provide feedback.

**Incorporate assessment in the initial planning**

Teachers need to look at how the outcome of learning will demonstrate student proficiency in the areas they are interested in. For example, if a teacher is interested in his/her students' improvement in oral skills then he/she could incorporate a video recording of students' presentations, which can be shared with the partner class. Clear criteria on what a good presentation means or entails can be discussed between the two groups. In the international online collaborative community health project (Sarr and Mason 2008); the evaluation of the exercises on identification of priority health issues was based on each group's performance on writing a proposal of identified priority health issues. The grading criteria focused on the above specific tasks that the groups in the two countries were required to carry out. Each group's proposal was limited to not more than 4 – 5 pages that justified its choice of priority health issues. After completing this exercise, students then engaged in discussions of the priority health issues identified in each country via email.

Written and oral reports were provided by student groups of their collaborative work and conclusions in both countries followed the exercise of comparing and contrasting priority health issues. Written reports were submitted for grading and disseminated (poster, Power Point presentations or other methods) among students in both countries during a final presentation to their respective classmates at both the University of The Gambia and the University of Miami.

Here, the assessment criteria focused on how based on their online discussion report student groups in each country summarised answers and conclusions to several questions on the identified health issues in the two different countries; the similarities and differences that exist in the countries, and solutions for each country's priority health issues. Students were expected to write reports that are clear, understandable, concise, and unambiguous with correct grammar and spelling.

For the oral report, the measures focused on students' clear summaries of the learning that occurred in their group regarding similarities and differences in public health issues, the group's proposed solution for each country's priority health issue, and presentation of information in a creative and professional manner.

**Get students to assemble examples of their own work**

Students' work can be evaluated by the teacher only on or between peers or self-assessed. Some ideas to conduct this in a fully participatory manner include:

- Assessment of the other group members anonymously that may include giving lower marks to anyone who is reported as not working by the majority of the group members.
- Voting by members to dismiss a student from the group, in which case the group member must find a way to participate or take a failing mark for the project.
- Teachers asking for random presentations of group work from different members of the group, so that anyone who is not collaborating will not be able to give a report.
- Using chat transcriptions, emails, etc

**Give guidelines to students for self and peer assessment**

Teachers can negotiate with the students the areas that will be assessed and discussed with them the various criteria that everyone agrees represent good standards. Components that teachers can include as guidelines for the assessment reports include:

- Preparation (collaboration)
- Participation (quality and quantity)
- Creativity (problem-solving)
- Contribution of ideas (collaboration)
- Punctuality (interpersonal skills)

- Respect (interpersonal skills)
- Commitment (collaboration)

**Think of using rubrics for measuring achievement**

Well-written rubrics (explanatory comments; headings or lines marked out in red) give a clear description of the levels of performance. It also helps the students to know what is expected of them. However, in order for the students to understand these expectations such rubrics must be provided with examples, such as giving samples taken from your students' work before the project began and using them to explain how to apply the rubrics. In addition, rubrics can assist the teacher

**Box 14 : Tips on writing rubrics that employ Bloom's Taxonomy in rubrics**

An assessment rubric is a matrix, grid or cross-tabulation employed with the intention of making expert judgments of student work both more systematic and more transparent to students. Rubrics explicate in summary form the bases upon which expert judgements are made. The rows set out the dimensions of the performance that have been selected as the aspects upon which the judgement will be focused. Each row corresponds to one dimension (aspect, property or characteristic) known as a criterion. Across the column heads of the matrix are set out the performance standards – typically four or five with labels indicative of each of the levels demonstrated (excellent, good, satisfactory, poor). Equivalently, a rubric may have its criteria listed as column headers and the standards as row labels. Ideally, the criteria are derived by analysing competent judgements about student performances to identify the dimensions that seem to explain the observed quality, and the standards set out the performance levels on those criteria. The information in the whole matrix is combined to arrive at an overall judgment of the quality of the student works.

**Example – essay**

Criteria that might be relevant include: structure of essay; clarity of expression; logic of the argument; and currency of the literature used. This list is not intended to be definitive – there could be more or fewer, similar or different criteria that are appropriate for particular tasks. Variation would normally be expected across disciplines and across year levels within a degree programme.

For each of the criteria in a rubric, various levels of performance could be described, either in general terms, or as specifics. As an example, consider the above case of the essay, and specifically the criterion Logic of the argument. Standards may be expressed in general terms such as Very poor; Poor; Mediocre; Good; and Excellent. Alternatively, specific descriptors may be developed and used: Mostly incoherent and difficult to follow; Weak progression of ideas and development; Moderately clear line of argument but with significant gaps; Ordered and basically logical; and Exemplary logical development throughout. Although in principle it may be appropriate to think of an underlying continuum of levels of performance, in practice that continuum is broken into a small number of ordinal categories (five in the example) that represent points along the quality continuum. In each of the intersecting cells of the rubric is entered the text that describes or characterises the quality of students' performance for the criterion (the row) at each standard (the column). After this is carried out for all the nominated criteria the whole is summarised for convenience as the rubric.

Completing the text-based description within the cells of a rubric can be challenging. It requires us to analyse and describe performances of various standards within each criterion. Some general models for classifying educational outcomes exist, and these can be useful in thinking through and articulating the achievement standards. One of the common models is the revised Bloom's taxonomy (Anderson & Krathwohl, 2001) which provides a logical sequence of learning development (remembering, understanding, applying, analysing, evaluating, creating) [Each element in the revised taxonomy has several key verbs associated with it:

- Remembering - recognising, listing, describing, identifying, retrieving, naming, locating, finding
- Understanding - interpreting, summarising, inferring, paraphrasing, classifying, comparing, explaining, exemplifying
- Applying - implementing, carrying out, using, executing
- Analysing - comparing, organising, deconstructing, attributing, outlining, finding, structuring, integrating
- Evaluating - checking, hypothesising, critiquing, experimenting, judging, testing, detecting, monitoring
- Creating - designing, constructing, planning, producing, inventing, devising, making]

This can provide useful triggers for thinking about a continuum of increasing complexity or sophistication of learning and its demonstration through assessment.

*Adapted from Smith et al (2013)*

organise the project because they clearly demonstrate the expected outcomes. The significance of this is that the teacher will have to plan carefully the tasks and project design in order to help the students reach the anticipated final products. Teachers can find tips and examples on writing rubrics that uses Bloom's Taxonomy (Bloom 1956) in rubrics via the Internet. Box 14 provides tips on writing rubrics that employs Bloom's Taxonomy in rubrics.

**You and your partner should take time to reflect on the experience**

Collaborative learning, like any new experience in teaching, takes some time for the student to feel comfortable with it and to feel that he/she really comprehends how to get the most out of the experience. Students' progress in such learning can be enhanced by sharing each other's reflections about how they feel the experience progresses and to provide your partner the same chance. Importantly, students should allow one another to express their opinions, whether positive or not, and maintain their focus on how to improve the project coordination and try to keep "personal" issues out of the evaluation.

An evaluation method used by Moen et al (2000) was adopted for the evaluation of the international online collaborative community health project. Quantitative and qualitative data were collected from student participants following the completion of the online assignment using a questionnaire. The questionnaire includes structured items and open-ended questions. Participants were provided with a hard copy of the questionnaire, which was written in English, the language understood by students in both countries.

Responses to the structured items were based on a 4-point Likert scale that ranged from strongly agree to strongly disagree, and a response category for neither agree nor disagree is included. Items addressed issues related to learning, interpersonal relationships, technology, and satisfaction. A score between 1 and 2.5 on each item on the 4-point scale was viewed as a positive result.

Qualitative data were collected from four sources. First, the questionnaire included seven open-ended questions that focused on what students considered meaningful. There were also probing questions on the responses to the structured items on the Likert scale. Second, a class discussion held at the end of the project allowed participants to debrief about the experience and offer recommendations about the process. Third, the transcripts of online dialogue were analysed; and fourth, the written assignments that were part of the project were reviewed and analysed using content analysis methods (Morgan 1993).

**Plan the final arrangements**

This is a creative process that requires participants who carry out various tasks to have some sort of "closing activity". This is necessary to assist students realise easily the benefits they get from the experience and are encouraged to participate in similar experiences in the future. It gives students the opportunity to look at the things they learnt, what they enjoyed, and how they think the project can be improved and to savour the personal benefit of having contacted partners they are not usually acquainted with. Moreover, such an activity has the merit of serving as a means for teachers to celebrate a positive experience or help diminish negative feeling about the project if things happen as anticipated (Dooly 2008).

**Points to remember about a good collaborative activity**

There are several important points to keep in mind:

- In carrying out their tasks students should be encouraged to reflect on how they came to their solutions of each problem they encountered.

• Students should learn to listen carefully to comments, opinions, suggestions and criticisms from other members of the group and learn to "re-think" their own judgments and opinions, when and if necessary. As mentioned in Part Two, Chapter 2, the collaborative learning activities should give students the chance to analyse, synthesise, and evaluate their ideas together. These higher order thinking skills serve as means to facilitate discussion and interaction that encourage students to progress beyond mere statements of opinion. Although network-based learning is a good way to design tasks that include ways of exchanging this information in groups, whether synchronously or asynchronously, the teacher should remember that the best method for exchanging information and opinions as well as the choice of ICT tool for doing this will rest on several contextual factors, such as the group personality, of which careful and active listening abilities is an important part.

**The task should lead to positive interdependence**

Needless to say, this is one of the most important factors to collaborative learning, as was evident in the international online collaborative health project. Students who know that each individual's participation is essential for the whole group can be highly motivated. This may require assigning each member of the group a different role; however, each role must be critical for the overall activity. Unavoidably, it may be necessary to conduct prompt and preliminary exercises in vocabulary and phrases for lower levels of language learners, but the students will have the chance to put this knowledge to use in authentic texts. It also allows the teacher (s) to distribute the tasks according to each student's individual abilities. Students who enjoy doing research can be assigned, for example, the role of conducting prompt and preliminary exercises in vocabulary and phrases; those who are much organised may be assigned to the role of reporter and so on, as indicated above. Such roles can also be rotated so that everyone has a chance to play a different role. Teachers should look for best strategies for promoting interdependence with their groups. Such strategies might include formulating tasks that compel students to reach a consensus, specifying common rewards for the group, and encouraging students to divide up the labour. The project helps the students develop effective interpersonal communication, which means that group members communicate with each other on a regular basis, and are careful to ensure that their communication is clear and relevant (Johnson et al 1987). This may depend on the ages of the students and the resources of the school such as teachers, class schedules and computer resources. If the students are older or more autonomous, then group collaboration may be the responsibility of the students themselves. Interpersonal communication, in this case, is essential and could even be deemed necessary for final assessment. Thus, both students and teachers should be trained in the various means of communication, such as online messenger services, e-mail and discussion boards, audio and video chats (Dooly 2008).

## Summary

In summary, this chapter has discussed aspects of a cooperative and collaborative project design with reference to building a community of learning in community health, giving examples and theoretical explanations from the education and community health literature and the writer's experience. First, the chapter outlined the significance of online collaborative and cooperative projects. Then it provided tips on how to come up with a good project idea. This is followed by steps to use during the planning, implementation and final stages. As already mentioned, teachers may find it difficult in ideal community health contexts to implement a full collaborative learning process in which students are completely autonomous and all the team members negotiate and decide the tasks or activities on their own. However, it can be a goal to strive for in community health. Thus, this chapter was aimed at helping those who wish to achieve the goal of designing online co-operative and collaborative learning projects in the community. What is clear from this and previous discussion is not only the importance of the role of the teacher in all the pedagogical, curricular and co-curricular processes described, but also the need for the link of teacher-professional development that enables teachers to carry out their roles most effectively, including training in the different means of communication that cooperative and collaborative learning requires.

The next two chapters deal with professional development opportunities that provide teachers with such development and teaching and learning centres that have much to do with teacher- professional development. As will be seen, both topics offer powerful mechanisms for stimulating institutional change that encompasses pedagogical, curricular, and co-curricular approaches. We will start with the chapter on professional development in community health.

# 12

## *Professional Development in Community Health*

Community health educators who experience professional development opportunities in the community value the opportunities that learning in the community offers (Bickford et al 2010)). Professional development refers to skills and knowledge attained for both personal development and career advancement. Professional development includes all types of facilitated learning opportunities, ranging from college degrees to formal coursework, conferences and informal learning opportunities situated in practice (such as semi-structured learning and occurs in a variety of places, such as learning at home, work, and through daily interactions and shared relationships among members of society). It has been described as intensive and collaborative, ideally incorporating an evaluative stage. There is a variety of similar but more specific and important approaches to professional development in community health education, such as consultation, coaching, communities of practice (see Part One Chapter 4 ), lesson study, mentoring, reflective supervision and technical assistance (e.g. Giri et al 2014)). For instance, Quinn (2000) describes how a community diagnosis course, an intensive field experience through which graduate students in health behaviour and health education conducted a community assessment, helped students in their development as community health educators.

According to Quinn, existing literature on the professional preparation of health educators and the writings of students who have completed the course demonstrate the professional skills that students gained through the experience. Students developed cultural competence, came to a more sophisticated understanding of their relationship to communities and their professional role as health educators. Cultural competence is considered one of the most promising tools for reducing the devastating effects of healthcare disparities resulting, as we have seen in Part 1, Chapter 1, from complex interacting factors, such as education, being uninsured, geography, poverty, gender, and racial and/or ethnic identity (NHDR, 2003). Betancourt et al (2002), for example, consider the use of organisational, systemic and clinical cultural competence as an urgent requirement for system change. Others (e.g. Mayberry et al. 2006) recommend that providers should carry out their tasks in a safe, timely, effective and efficient manner. This should be done with equity and the practice of patient centredness – a goal that could be achieved through cultural competence.

There are various definitions of cultural competence. The Office of Minority Health (NCMHD 2008) defines cultural competence as "....a set of congruent behaviours, attitudes, and policies that come together in a system, agency, or among professionals that enables effective work in cross-cultural situations." Other meanings of cultural competence acknowledge significance aspects such as humility, cultural sensitivity, effectiveness and responsiveness (Betancourt et al. 2003). However, all the definitions share the fundamental requirements for providers to be sensitized to their patients by adjusting their own cultures to understand those of their patients (Johnson et al. 2004). If healthcare workers understand the sociological and cultural factors that influence patients' beliefs and behaviours and how they interact at multiple levels (i.e. organisational, structural and clinical) to affect decision making, they will be able to design intervention techniques to improve healthcare treatment and delivery outcomes (e.g. Ngo-Metzger et al. 2006). The goal of cultural competence is to develop a culturally competent workforce and healthcare system for delivering the best quality of care possible to patients in spite of language ability, race, ethnicity or culture.

The students gained experience working effectively as part of a team, and learn specific skills in conducting needs assessments, gathering and analysing qualitative and quantitative data, and building collaborative efforts. This example shows that efforts are being made in community health education to identify training and personal development needs and to design programmes that provide professional development opportunities for community health practitioners and their employers.

However, as we will see later in this and the following chapter, much of such innovations do not adequately meet the needs of primary health care/community health education. First, this chapter considers how community health educators and their partners can identify relevant curriculum content for professional development in community health, emphasising content that meets the needs of community health education in the 21st century. The chapter finally looks at needed changes in health care and education systems in support of professional development in community health education.

## Identifying Professional Development Needs

We must start by making two points which may be clear or implied in the discussion so far. One is that professional development in community health does not only consist of traditional training which is required to cover essential work-related skills, techniques and knowledge, but most importantly it also enables learning and personal development, which the above examples show and chapters in Part One have dealt with in some detail. As we have seen, learning and personal development extend the range of development way outside conventional work skills and knowledge, and creates far more exciting, liberating, motivational opportunities for people and for employers. As we mentioned earlier, healthcare systems are increasingly becoming more complex and changing rapidly. Consequently, organisations in health care are facing great pressure to change to meet the demands of professional development in order to facilitate and encourage development and fulfilment of the whole person in addition to traditional training. The second point is that community health educators should use curriculum planning models and approaches that can adequately accommodate the realities that account for the limitations in PHC and community-oriented education and practice. These realities include especially social, political and economic factors, and other related factors that influenced health care in the past three decades, are doing so now and will do so in the future. We start with the business of identifying professional development needs through training needs analysis.

**Training Needs Analysis**

To be effective in identifying professional development needs a training needs analysis should identify those who need training and the type of training required to avoid training opportunities being offered to individuals who do not need them, or the wrong kind of training being provided. A training needs analysis will also assist in identifying training resources and putting them to good use. Let us now look at methods that can be used in training needs analysis.

**Types of Training Needs Analysis**

There are several training needs assessments that community health educators can use in various health service and education contexts. The features of sources that can assist educators determine which needs analysis is suitable for their situations are outlined below:

Organisational Analysis: An analysis of the business needs or other reasons the training is desired; an analysis of the organisation's strategies, goals, and objectives. The important questions being answered by this analysis are:

- What is the organisation overall trying to accomplish?
- Who decided that training should be conducted?
- Why is a training programme seen as the recommended solution to a business problem?
- What has been the history of the organisation with regard to employee training and other management interventions?

Person Analysis: Analysis dealing with potential participants and instructors involved in the process. The important questions being answered by this analysis are:

- Who will receive the training and their level of existing knowledge on the subject?
- What is their learning style, and who will conduct the training?
- Do the employees have the required skills?
- Are there changes to policies, procedures, software, or equipment that require or necessitate training?

Work analysis / Task Analysis: Analysis of the tasks being performed. This is an analysis of the job and the requirements for performing the work. It is also known as a task analysis or job analysis. The important question being answered by this analysis is:

What are the main duties and skill level required?

Performance Analysis: This helps ensure that the training which is developed will include relevant links to the content of the job. The important questions being asked by this analysis are:

- Are the employees performing up to the established standard?
- If performance is below expectations, can training help to improve this performance?
- Is there a Performance Gap?

Content Analysis: Analysis of documents, laws, procedures used on the job. This analysis answers questions about:

- What knowledge or information is used on this job?

  This information comes from manuals, documents, or regulations. It is important that the content of the training does not conflict or contradict job requirements. An experienced worker can assist (as a subject-matter expert) in determining the appropriate content.

  Training Suitability Analysis: It is an analysis of whether training is the desired solution. Training is one of several solutions to employment problems. However, it may not always be the best solution. The important question being asked by this analysis is:
- Is training the best solution to the service or work problems?

  Cost-Benefit Analysis: It is an analysis of the return on investment (ROI) of training. The important question being asked by this analysis is:
- Will effective training results in a return of value to the organisation that is greater than the initial investment to produce or administer the training (HR-Survey.com (2013)

These methods can identify those who need training and what kind of training is needed. These methods, as we can see in Part One, Chapter 3, are consistent mainly with the objectives model (see also the subject-centred curriculum model) which is useful in the area of training and suitable in the provision of instructions. But as we have seen, the objectives model, among other things, focuses on skills and knowledge acquisition only. Higher order thinking skills, problem solving and values development are important educational functions that could not be written in behavioural terms that is linked to the objectives model. This is indeed an important consideration when identifying learning and personal development needs that extend the range of development way outside conventional work skills and knowledge, and creates far more exciting, liberating, motivational opportunities for people and for employers. To achieve these important educational and service outcomes, we need other approaches for identifying such learning and personal development needs. More specifically, we need the descriptive and open-ended kinds of curriculum planning models outlined in Part One, Chapter 3 that can incorporate these critical outcomes, as well as provide community health educators a framework for accommodating health realities (economic, social, environmental, political and cultural factors, see Part One, Chapter 1) in their planning for community health. One of such curriculum planning models – cultural analysis model- can be a useful approach to identifying learning and personal development needs in particular, as well as the educational needs for promoting community health.

**Cultural Analysis Approach**

As already mentioned, cultural analysis is a method by which course planners can analyse the culture of a society - the social (which includes political and health systems), economic, technology, communication, belief, morality and aesthetic systems of culture (Lawton (1983) - to obtain a clear picture of the factors health professionals confront. Course planners can identify learning and personal development needs that are more relevant to community health, by using a cultural analysis approach. Cultural analysis allows for the incorporation of other educational models, for example, the curriculum process model and other concepts, principles and scenarios to guide course planners (Lawton 1983), as well as policy-makers and other stakeholders in related professional development planning processes.

The cultural analysis curriculum planning approach is, firstly, a method of education and is therefore applicable to planning education for all health professionals - doctors, nurses, dentists, etc., trained persons who help in identifying or preventing or treating illness or disability. Secondly, based on a wider view of education, it is flexible and open enough to accommodate important educational proposals in community health, such as interdisciplinary education. If the success required in this and other important areas of learning is to be achieved, the educational needs that health professionals have in common must be planned together by curriculum planners in the different health professions, through a common curriculum. The common curriculum idea demands that curriculum planners decide on the concepts and experiences which will give access to worthwhile knowledge (see curriculum process model, Part One, Chapter 3) and make it possible for all students to access this minimum programme. Some students will certainly progress much further, while some will fall behind in the basic understanding of the common curriculum programme (Lawton 1983).

However, all students will have been given access to useful knowledge (Lawton 1982). This proposal is the subject of another book by the author entitled *Community-Oriented Education for Health Professional: Cultural Analysis Approach to Curriculum Planning* (Sarr 2013), in which he justifies this suggestion. In 2008, after more than 30 years of Primary Health Care (PHC) policy coming from the Alma Ata Declaration there have been calls for a renewal of PHC. For example, the World Health Report 2008 (WHO 2008) and the Report of the Commission on the Social Determinants of Health (Peters et al 2009) reaffirmed the relevance of PHC in terms of its vision and values in today's world. However, such calls for the renewal of the policy are not without commentary on the results. Member states of the WHO agreed that with even 30 years of implementing PHC health systems still do not advance optimal care due to their failure to promote an appropriate balance in their efforts in terms of disease prevention, health promotion, cure and palliative care (WHO 2008).

Similarly, important challenges have been identified by others. For instance, in an article that reviews developments in the last 32 years and discusses the future of PHC policy Bhatia et al (2010) put forward three challenges for discussion. They are (i) the challenge of moving away from a narrow technical bio-medical paradigm of health to a broader social determinants approach and the need to differentiate primary care from primary health care (ii) the challenge of tackling the equity implications of the market-oriented reforms and ensuring that the role of the State in the provision of welfare services is not further weakened (iii) the challenge of finding ways to develop local community commitments especially in terms of empowerment. They suggest that these challenges need to be addressed if PHC is to remain relevant in today's context, and conclude that it is not sufficient to revitalise PHC of the Alma Ata Declaration but it must be reframed in light of the above discussion.

As mentioned in the publication, such pressing challenges are characterised by enormously high complexity. Depending on past experience to decide what to do is no longer adequate. There is need to find new ways to solve problems that provide opportunities to discover innovations that have the potential to bring about a better and more promising future. The way we think and do things needs to change from closed to open, from mere debating to reflective and generative dialogue, and from an autocratic leadership model to one of shared or collective leadership. But most importantly, there is need to have the will to change one's self before one can change the system. As managers of healthcare institutions and leaders to other healthcare providers, it is in the interest of health professionals (and others concerned), not only to take on these challenges, but also to get to grips with them-as far as their capabilities allow.

This requires planners of educational programmes for health professionals to use curriculum planning models that can adequately accommodate in particular the social, political, economic and other realities or factors that influenced health care. Indeed, the Network of Community-oriented Institutions for the Health Sciences (Schmidt et al 1991) that was created at the instigation of the WHO and whose main aim is to provide mutual support to member institutions that desire to adapt their curricula to the health needs of the communities they serve, has revealed that one of the lessons it has learnt in its ten years of existence is that "a more precise analysis of the political and socio-economic environments within which the schools operate is necessary for achieving the desired goal of producing physicians who will contribute to the health of individuals and communities," (Schmidt et al 1991, p 262).

This is because in many countries the existing realities of the healthcare delivery system significantly influence the ultimate performance of students, probably more than the types or quality of the education they receive in the schools. In fact, it was through analysis of the underlying social, economic and political causes of ill health that the report of the Commission on Social Determinants of Health (Peters et al 2009) made a case for and supported the renewal of the PHC policy. Thus, from a health professional education perspective, one can draw strong justification from these and many similar experiences for providing health professional opportunities for understanding such realities in health care and developing the skills necessary to deal with them with the aim of enhancing the PHC policy. Such experiences must constitute the most important aspects of professional development programmes with a community health centric focus.

Not much has been said so far about how curriculum planners can identify curriculum content in community health schools for the pre-service education of health professionals for the community. But curriculum planners in such schools need to be also guided if they are to be successful in such undertaking. The cultural analysis planning framework provides curriculum planners a tool for identifying relevant curriculum content with productive learning experiences that can accommodate the realities to meet the needs of community health education.

The cultural analysis approach has the distinct advantage that curriculum planners can address in their planning all the interrelated eight systems or characteristics that all societies have in common for the education of healthcare professionals for the community. Its use for such planning is based on the premise that it is impossible to train and educate adequately health professionals for the community which is perplexing and constantly differentiating unless understanding of the eight features is included in their education and training, in which their professional development is an important part.

Using this approach, community health educators can identify training and development needs that agree with the two distinct elements of the model of developed carrier practice within the community outlined by Boaden et al (1999) in discussing education for community practice. In this book, professional development is discussed within the domain of continuing education, as Boaden et al have seemingly done, and so their views on continuing education are relevant to this discussion on professional development in community health. One element is the necessity for health professionals to develop and maintain the aspect of core practice which will continue to be their role. While the boundaries of this role may change, it is not likely that many activities will do so. But the knowledge base and skills used in providing those core functions and the attitudes of patients receiving care will change. There will be the need to develop the personal qualities that make up an important part of community both in relation to patients and those who care for them, as well as the members of the complex primary healthcare teams which are evolving. Professionals will need to develop skills that are less concerned with detailed medical knowledge, for instance, and are more involved with interactive skills and broader knowledge of the sources of stress as well as the community resources that can be provided to deal with them. Connected to this are the personal components of professional development, such as portfolio learning, mentoring and the outcomes of small group learning are means by which these issues can be addressed. So also is the need for development of professional skills for community practice, audit, research and the ability to deal with change within practice and in practice environments.

Simultaneously, parallel to these core roles will be additional new roles health professional have to play which stem from the much wider view involved in the more developed kinds of community-based practice. Although economic arguments will encourage such changes, there will also be professional arguments for changes in the definition of roles and the joining of various professional skills within health teams. Needless to say, the establishment of community-based healthcare teams means that greater specialisation will be expected.

Boaden et al (1999) suggest that the non-core development and innovatory practice area is where the community-based health care of the future has to develop. Functions in this area include advocacy in the community, research and development, management and participation in healthcare teams and proactive population-based practice. They argue that while some of these functions fall within the present undergraduate programmes, evidently the coverage provided in these programmes is not sufficient enough to prepare professionals to meet the challenges of the future.

The cultural analysis planning framework provides curriculum planners a tool for identifying relevant curriculum content in these areas of professional development in the community. Selection from the analysis of the eight systems of culture ( Part One, Chapter 3) in the context of community health in a particular country, The Gambia, for example (as described in Sarr (2013), has shown in brief that it is important to stress in the curriculum of health professionals knowledge of the significance of personal values, beliefs in health care and understanding of the importance of socio-cultural factors in disease prevention. This must be accompanied by relevant applied science and mathematics, including psychosocial science and political science. The common curriculum should include people's moral thinking and feeling about health and diseases. The delivery of PHC that is meaningful, acceptable, accessible, effective and cost–effective demands a better understanding of the socio-cultural backgrounds of patients and clients, their families and the environment in which they live. It is crucial to have a good knowledge of how peoples' cultural values, beliefs and assumptions influence the care provided and are formed by social relationships and the context in which health workers live and work. It further demonstrates that the eight systems of cultural analysis are closely interrelated. For example, the social, communication and technology systems are clearly connected to one another and to the aesthetic system in terms of the aspects of communication and technology that can be used in both simple and complex aesthetic experiences to tackle socio-cultural, patient care and other issues in health care. Pertinent knowledge of these should be important parts of a common curriculum. As in the communication and technology systems, the effective use of simple and complex or modern aesthetic experiences in health care requires inter- and intra-sectoral collaboration and pertinent decisions and actions with respect to health policy, reward systems, expenditure patterns, distribution of resources, etc.

In addition to development in these core and non-core areas, community health educators must improve in the curriculum development endeavour. The development of professional development programmes and the use of the relatively novel teaching and learning modes that will be required to implement them will make particular demands on the expertise and skills of teachers, among other things, and the responsibility of the leader of community health educators in developing teachers and others concerned (clinical staff, supervisors, etc) cannot be overstated. Perhaps nowhere is the saying that there cannot be effective curriculum development without teacher development truer than in the business of planning a cultural analysis and PHC/Community Health-type professional development programmes. The leader must provide the opportunities that will ensure that the necessary skills and expertise are developed or reinforced through school – based and community-based professional development programmes. They must, in particular, be prepared for the new roles the integrated curriculum, the process curriculum model, problem-solving and multi-professional approaches, together with the new teaching/learning principles, strategies and approaches, particularly cooperative and collaborative learning, as well synchronous and asynchronous learning, will create.

The significance of such professional development becomes clearer when it is looked at, for instance, in relation to the curriculum process model which, as mentioned earlier, rests on teacher judgment rather than on teacher direction. It is far more demanding on teachers and therefore far more difficult to implement in practice (although it offers a high degree of personal and professional development). There are also difficulties in assessment of students that the process model poses, such as exposure of the strengths and weaknesses of teachers (Stenhouse 1975). This calls for development of the teacher's skills and understanding of the concept so that he or she can appreciate the value of the curriculum process concept and be able and willing to participate actively in its implementation, including assessment on which it is based. The same applies to the concepts of the integrated curriculum, common curriculum, the problem-solving approach, and education for work.

The knowledge and skills of teachers must be developed in terms of awareness of the characteristics of these concepts and the behaviour needed for their implementation. This must include not only knowledge about the concepts and skills for using them, but also social and political skills such as negotiation, cooperation, advocacy, lobbying, etc – skills that are absent in many training curricula of health professionals that have been identified using the cultural analysis framework (Sarr 2013). The aim of such professional development should be to enable the teachers to influence decisions that can bring about changes in structural arrangements, expenditure patterns, organisational, and administrative structures that are needed for implementing the change effectively. For example, the task of scheduling several large classes of students into a technology laboratory with inadequate seats is an example of the problems associated with insufficiency of physical resources that requires considerable negotiating patience and skill on the part of teachers and the team leader.

Indeed, in many agencies that were responsible for initiating change, the most crucial influence on success was that the head teacher (or other members of the faculty ) had undertaken courses on, for example, leadership and managing change. Such courses were responsible for providing the initial impetus for some of the innovations (e.g. Gordon et al 1998). Such professional development, like curriculum development, must be school or community-based. As such they provide the leader and his/her team opportunities for linking closely curriculum development with teacher development, and development of their collaborators. It is therefore preferred to sending, for example, staff abroad for curriculum development-related further education. However, in order to facilitate strategy formulation the leader and his/her team can also consider the need for new ways of thinking in curriculum planning and, thus, the necessity of sending managers or other members of the team abroad or to other places outside community health schools sometimes to gain new perspectives (e.g. Gordon et al 1998). The identification of such training and development needs by community health educators using the approaches outlined above is a useful first step in a uniform method of programme design not only for pre-service education for health professionals but also for especially their professional development for community health practice. We present a few examples of professional development programme designs.

It is apparent from the foregoing discussion that efforts are being made in community health education to identify training and learning as well as personal development needs and to design programmes that provide professional development opportunities for community health practitioners and their employers. But community health educators and their partners must ensure that such efforts focus primarily and more seriously on meeting the needs of primary health care/community health. As we have seen, it is necessary for medical professionals, for example, to develop and maintain the aspect of core practice which will continue to be their role in the community. They will need to develop skills that are less concerned with detailed medical knowledge and are more involved with interactive skills and broader knowledge of the sources of stress as well as the community resources that can be provided to deal with them. Most importantly, with regard to the non-core development and innovatory practice area professionals will need to improve skills in, for instance, advocacy in the community, research and development, management and participation in healthcare teams and proactive population-based practice.

In addition to development in these core and non-core areas, community health educators must also be developed in the curriculum development endeavour that entails not only improving skills for the development of professional development programmes that address these concerns, but also the use of the relatively novel teaching and learning modes that will be required to implement them. As already mentioned, Boaden et al (1999) argue that even where some of these functions are covered in present undergraduate programmes, evidently the coverage provided in these programmes is not adequate enough to prepare professionals to meet the challenges in community health of the future. This is because of the conservative approach to present innovation by professionals that makes effecting change within health training institutions and healthcare systems difficult. Thus, the need for a change in attitude and the manner we plan and manage the many educational innovations in the community. Boaden et al suggest several needed changes in healthcare and education systems which the following section outlines.

**Required Changes in Healthcare and Educational Systems**

This section describes some of the important changes that are required in relation to non-core development, structures for professional development, learning organisations, support for professional development, accreditation, and career transition in community-based practice.

**Non-core Development**

- Proper resourcing used to enable the practice organisation to create the space and time for facilitation of effective study, not for rewarding the practitioner.
- Changes in the management and organisation of practice that will increase the demand and provision of professional development.
- Making professional development inter-professional because future practice and future practice needs mirror this model.

**Structures for Professional Development**

- Bringing education and practice closer together in the context of professional development. Practice requires to be organised to suit the needs of provision of future care, as well as facilitation of the kind of education professional will require for such care.
- Creating an educational system planned to provide such education and to meet the demands that health professions will have to deal with in the new system. This requires (i) that both the healthcare and professional education must be interdisciplinary in nature and bring together the different agencies involved in the community using approaches that enhance practice and education for practice and (ii) both must give the right environment for planning, managing and resourcing education and practice effectively.
- Educational reform must anticipate changes in practice and lead them to enhance efficient and effective change.

**Learning Organisations**

- Providing health professionals greater opportunities for experiential learning. This requires the organisations involved in and linked to health care to provide innovative services as well as create a conducive environment for professional development.
- Both organisation and health professionals must be able to initiate change and innovate the working practices and new treatments and preventive strategies made possible by the new healthcare arrangement.
- Providing basic learning chances concerning the work that has not been covered in initial professional training and education.
- The process of mentoring, portfolio learning, etc., which are traditionally undertaken with fellow professionals in learning core skills must be pro-

vided in the work setting of the community in line with current views about how health professionals should be trained for roles in community health.

**Accreditation**

- Accreditation of community health practitioners is needed to establish credibility of the developing community-based practice, particularly to the extended concept of that practice.
- Establishing a system to accredit practitioners requires (i) establishing standards of performance which can be measured and which reflect the outcome of the activity instead of the activity itself (ii) including the new disciplines and their contribution in the system (iii) guaranteeing minimum standards using a process that encourages the search for better standards and improving practice (iv) establishing a system to handle the process of accreditation.
- Including peer-review in the process although this by itself may not be a sufficient guarantee of performance.
- Including audit and research in the nature of community-based practice, as well as sharing information between professionals and agencies involved.
- Extending accreditation not only to health professionals but also to organisations involved.

**Career transitions in community-based practice**

- Career transition within community-based practice which requires preparation of the health professional include some taking on the supervisory role with staff who may be given increased autonomy, but whose position may not deserve overall independent practice.
- It includes someone taking responsibility for training of staff within the team, and to deal with the development of teamwork which is consistent with the new kind of community-based practice. (Boaden et al 1999)

**Summary**

This chapter considered how curriculum planners can identify relevant curriculum content for professional development that meets the needs of community health now and in the future. Then it outlined needed changes in healthcare and educational systems in support of professional development. The business of identifying professional development needs for community health education should be conducted at school, departmental and community levels and must involve all teachers and other stakeholders concerned. Although time-consuming, the techniques described can be useful for updating existing professional development programmes and designing new ones for community health practitioners.

The following chapter deals with the task of developing teaching and learning centres that provide opportunities for professional development and can serve as settings that promote a community of learning for community health, as well as offering powerful mechanisms for stimulating institutional change that encompasses pedagogical, curricular, and co-curricular approaches.

# 13

## *Development of Teaching and Learning Centres in Community Health*

This chapter deals with the issue of developing teaching and learning centres in community health education. First, the chapter outlines various types of teaching and learning centres in both developed and developing countries. It then focuses on the development of teaching and learning centres that are best suited to the needs of community health/PHC education, placing emphasis on TLCs (Teaching and Learning Centres) that are located in decentralised systems of PHC. Finally, the chapter describes a teaching and learning centre design strategy that is consistent with the concepts and principle of community health/PHC and is appropriate to local circumstances.

**Types of Teaching and Learning Centres**

The wealth of information from the literature shows that the term teaching and learning centres are commonly used in mainly developed countries within colleges and universities or their partner institutions to describe centres that provide professional development or continuing education in a variety of disciplines (e.g. CQ University 2011). Like the professional development approaches reported in the education and community health literature, teaching and learning centres including those that focus on the community are as diverse in their aims and ownership as they vary in their definitions, methods and approaches to such education. For example, there are teaching and learning centres in developed countries (e.g. University of Melbourne 2013) where the aim is to provide general practice education for medical students through clinical placements in general practice and give GPs professional development opportunities in clinical supervision which is a typical service that TLCs offer. There are also TLCs that provide professional development/continuing education in developed countries other than TLCs located in universities/colleges or affiliated institutions. For instance, in several

European countries government organisations, municipal organisations, foundations and associations, voluntary and charity organisations, Non-Governmental Organisations, local public centres (libraries), commercial learning institutes and companies (in-house training) also provide professional development/continuing education in local learning centres (LLCs) that are defined as any initiative that includes local learning (European Commission DG 2005). However, in these countries there are also great variations in aims, methods and terminology used to describe teaching and learning centres.

Similarly, in Asia and Pacific countries there are various types of community learning centres (CLCs) and terms used to describe them. Some CLCs are supported by governments, some by NGOs and donors, while others are fully owned and managed by communities. There are also adult/youth literacy centres which were designed after CLC concepts and approaches and which currently function like CLCs (UNESCO 2012). Also, such lack of uniformity in terminology, function, support and ownership of TLCs are found in other parts of the world, such as Africa and South Pacific countries like Australia where TLCs that have a community health/PHC focus have been called Primary Healthcare Academic Centres or Academic Primary Healthcare sites.

**Community Health/PHC-Oriented Teaching and Learning Centres**

Here again, like in the discussion on professional development, it is worth stating an issue that must be a major consideration in establishing teaching and learning centres that are suited to community health needs. As already mentioned, the conservative approach to present innovations in community-based medical education, for example, is pushed by limited objectives and outcomes from the medical professional framework. This approach uses a simplified primary care model of community-based health care that poses difficulties in implementing change, both within the institutions of medical education and across the structures of health care with their enduring entrenched patterns of professional dominance and relatively poor in-agency and inter-professional cooperation (Boaden et al 1999). As we indicated, this requires not only a change in attitude, but also changes in the way we plan and manage the many educational innovations in the community. In proposing changes in healthcare and education system to address issues in continuing education/professional development, Boaden et al reveal that there are centres that focus on developing the skills of facilitators and teachers from the new subject areas involved in community-based practice of their knowledge of the health service through research and consultancy which can inform their education and training roles and make them convey confidence and respect.

However, the character of such centres is limited in scope and at times provides a model of provision which is expensive and cannot be easily used by practitioners that require the service they provide (ibid). Boaden et al (1999) also inform that the services the centres provide are oriented around the institutional norms of higher education (where, as the literature shows, teaching and learning centres (TLCs) are mainly located in developed countries) involving formal qualifications and the structure of provision corresponding with the traditional demands of such qualifications. Such facilities are also used by the minority of practitioners, or by those who have to wait for their turn, be given study leave and have the needed time for study. As they suggest, community-based practice needs a different approach that involves distance learning that allows practitioners to attend periodically local facilities to give the needed contact which is often not possible with formal courses, access to educational material organised in a way that facilitates use and short courses.

This need for a different approach to developing TLCs which is now greatly encouraged by, for example, the drive to extend the range of disciplines relevant to community-based practice as required by the PHC principles is generating other attempts to developing teaching and learning centres in various countries. But perhaps nowhere is the needed change in approach more evident than in African countries that have long adopted the PHC strategy. As we have seen in Part One, Chapter 1, the educational focus to the community that is driven by the PHC principles and the resultant educational gains are much more noticeable in these developing countries that have for many years embraced the PHC approach and have been able to express its principles practically in the education process than in developed countries.

For instance, the Western Cape Community Partnership Project in Cape Town, South Africa, has developed Academic Primary Healthcare Sites, the goal of which is to contribute to significant education of health professionals through stemming the decline in the number of graduates selecting PHC and increasing the number of health professionals better educated and dedicated to primary healthcare practice in community settings. The stakeholders see this goal as being consistent with the concept of community-based education (CBE) as an outcome of developing educational methods in general and in higher education especially. At the learning sites PHC and CBE are seen as an approach to health development involving the total orientation of the health system with these features: the participation of the community, greater equitable distribution of health resources, giving more to primary health care and its supervisory level, and enhancing health prevention, promotion and rehabilitative care; orientation of the health services to enable secondary and tertiary care to support care at primary care level (which is the first level of contact) therefore involving the total health system, and inter-sectoral coordination.

Use of this comprehensive PHC approach is limited in the TLCs of many countries in terms of their scope, aims, methods and approaches. It is clear that the activities of many TLCs are still conditioned by the primary care model which reflects, as Boaden et al suggest, the relatively modest objectives that arise within the well-established professional framework which adopts a relatively narrow primary care model of community-based health care. This, as indicated earlier, while being an essential subset of primary health care and complementary with it, deals mainly with the prevention and treatment of sickness. It is what many people think of as front-line care. Conventionally, this takes the form of a visit to the family doctor. Primary care may involve preventative activities, immunisation, diagnosis and treatment of illness. But such a care usually does not include a comprehensive, inter-sectoral approach to producing or enhancing health. Perhaps most crucially, primary care concentrates on individuals and families, but not the community as the unit of intervention which is one of the hallmarks of the primary healthcare approach.

The vision of this new approach is to create a community health-centric, comprehensive, accessible and flexible system to make teaching and learning centre management processes more effective and efficient. The following sections will present a description of a project design to meet this vision in the community. The system holds promise for a streamlined management of professional development/continuing education in community health. As already indicated, design is the creation of a plan for the construction of an object or a system; an organisational arrangement, or structure of elements, parts, or details.

In Part Two, Chapter 1, we suggested that learning space in the community should be designed to support a community of learners. We presented several tips for undertaking new capital learning space design projects in the community, pointing out how these tips can be applied in building a community of learning for community health and giving theoretical explanations and examples from the relevant literature. This includes designing capital learning space projects in teaching and learning centres at the different local levels of health care that have a community health-centric mission. Such a construction project, as we have seen, produces a complex system with human and mechanical components and the value generated by the project is embedded in the system. Here, TLC projects produce a desired change in systems or processes of professional development/continuing education in community health. Such projects are also meant to produce an operationally effective process in such professional development/continuing education. This chapter looks at the strategy for the development of such projects that must also consider the principles, approaches and good practices in any design process of a development intervention we outlined in previous discussions.

## Design Strategy

As in learning space and pedagogical, curricular and co-curricular designs, it is particularly crucial to involve stakeholders in teaching and learning centre design to ensure the design strategy is appropriate to local circumstances. With several groups of stakeholders a situation analysis is conducted to learn as much as possible about the project context and the interests and needs of local people in order to design a relevant project. Recent studies and leading management theorists have advocated that strategy needs to start with stakeholders' expectations and use a modified balanced scorecard which includes all stakeholders. While not always required, design strategy often uses social research methods to help ground the results and mitigate the risk of any course of action. The approach has proved useful for companies in a variety of strategic scenarios. As can be seen in Part Two, Chapter 1, on learning space design, paying careful attention to the social processes and institutional development that will enable learning and the empowerment of primary stakeholders, as well as carrying out a detailed situation analysis with stakeholders are considered important requirements of the design process.

One result of a good situation analysis is that stakeholders have more insights about their situation and have better capacity to design a solid project. With a good understanding of the situation, one is now ready to start developing the design strategy. This simply explains clearly what everyone hopes to achieve, why do it and how it will be achieved, how to innovate contextually, both immediately and over the long term. This process involves the interplay between design and business strategy, forming a systematic approach integrating holistic-thinking and research methods used to inform business strategy and strategic planning which provides a context for design. Business strategy (Strategic Management) analyses the major initiatives taken by a community health school's top management and collaborating partners on behalf of owners, involving resources and performance in community settings. It involves describing the organisation's mission, vision and objectives, developing policies and plans, often in terms of projects and programmes, which are designed to achieve these objectives, and then allocating resources to implement the policies, plans, projects and programmes. A balanced scorecard is often used to evaluate the overall performance of the business and its progress towards objectives. The balanced scorecard is a strategy performance management tool - a semi-standard structured report, supported by design methods and automation tools that can be used by community health education managers to keep track of the execution of activities by the staff within their control and to monitor the consequences arising from these actions.

Design strategy can play an integral role in helping to resolve common problems in developing teaching and learning centres plans in the community. One common problem is identifying the most important questions that a teaching and learning centre in the community should address. Another common problem is promoting the adoption of a technology, such as the ICTs used in synchronous and asynchronous learning, as well as cooperative and collaborative learning (Chapter 9). There is the need to connect design efforts to a teaching and learning centre's business strategy, which focuses most intently on designs that simplify technology experiences and results in lower manufacturing costs at a time when health systems are pushing for cost-cutting. There is the question of how to translate insights into actionable solutions in the complex and increasing changing communities in health care. There is also the issue of prioritising the order in which plans should be launched, whether plans should be launched slowly over time, rather than launching all of its components at once.

Thus, designing teaching and learning centres plans, like developing curricular, and co-curricular plans, should also parallel the learning space design which strongly affects the facilitation of the execution of teaching and learning centres' plans, programmes and projects subsequently via, for instance, the relationships and commitment established with partners and local people, particularly the intended primary stakeholders; the logic and feasibility of the development strategy; the resources allocated to teaching and learning centres (funding, time, expertise); the degree of inbuilt flexibility that allows teaching and learning centre plans to have an operational function; any operational details of the teaching and learning centre plans that might be established during initial design.

Like in the design of pedagogical, curricular, and co-curricular plans, a broad teaching and learning centre framework should be developed to provide: a) sufficient detail to enable budgeting and allocation of technical expertise, b) an overview of how teaching and learning centres plans will be implemented, and c) some guidance for all involved about how teaching and learning centre plans should be developed. We will now look at these and other related issues in more detail (e.g. IFAD 2011)

**Project goal**

This should reflect the longer-term and highest-level impact to which the project will contribute. Here the design team should not define overly ambitious goal or purposes, given local conditions and available resources and capacities. They must not overlook key activities and outputs that are needed to achieve higher-level objectives (outcomes/purpose/goal). The logic as to why particular activities are needed for a certain output or particular outputs for a certain purpose must be good. Objectives should be expressed clearly, precisely, and simply in order to know what will be achieved or how to implement ideas. Be it as it may, a teaching and learning centre with a community health centric-mission must have goals that are consistent with the principles and elements of PHC and the cooperative and collaborative learning modes that can foster a community of learning for community health. An example of such goal is:

> *…to contribute to the significant change of educating health professionals by adding to the number of health professionals who value learning and working cooperatively and collaboratively and are better educated and dedicated to the practice of community health/PHC in community settings (Adapted from Seth 1998, p.41)*

Not only will the achievement of such a goal increase the relevance of teaching and learning centres in the community, their realisation will also introduce novel ideas in community-oriented education that will help relate more closely the education of health professionals to the problems of society as required by the PHC approach. This calls for the kinds of professional development opportunities that the previous chapter dealt with and will be further considered in a following section on the activities of the teaching and learning centres.

**Purpose(s)**

This is what must be achieved by the project in order to contribute to the goal. The purpose level generally describes major changes in behaviour or capacity. Because a project can contribute to the goal in many ways, community health educators and other stakeholders will need to decide what is most worthwhile and feasible for designing teaching and learning centre plans, programmes and projects. The purpose helps to establish criteria to help make these decisions. As we have seen, generally, teaching and learning centres are independent academic units within colleges and universities. These centres may have different kinds of names, such as faculty development centres, teaching and learning centres, centres for teaching and learning, centres for teaching excellence, academic support centres, and others. Teaching and learning centres include experimental classrooms, consultation, and evaluation of student learning. Teaching and learning centres may exist to:

- provide support services for faculty, to help teaching faculty to improve their teaching and professional development.
- provide learning support services for students, and other services, depending on the individual institution.
- provide strong mechanisms for stimulating institutional change that encompasses pedagogical, curricular, and co-curricular approaches.
- advance partnerships between student development and faculty.
- prepare faculty to facilitate learning in community.
- help instructors to modernise their teaching style, to scaffold concepts and information in a way that students can meaningfully take in, and to help students learn more deeply and retain what they have learned. As such, these centres assume roles as educational change agents.
- attempt to help instructors with other problems that they might have, such as managing graduate students, designing courses, technical writing, trying novel teaching methods, and designing better assignments and exams.
- address learning difficulties at the students' end, by providing support services for better learning and study skills. Now many centres may also be involved in e-learning and similar movements.

As the foregoing discussion in Chapter 12 and this chapter suggest, these are common intentions of many university/college-based teaching and learning centres in developed countries including universities/colleges whose mission include healthcare education. For example, in one university in the US (Ukaigwe 2013) the teaching and learning centre manages educational programmes in a variety of disciplines including courses on global health. The TLC provides mainly professional development and supports faculty and students. For instance, teachers write courses and give to the TLC to put on Blackboard to allow students to review (syllabus, lectures, links, etc.) information on their own schedule. Blackboard is a tool that allows faculty to add resources for students to access online. PowerPoint, Captivate, video, audio, animation, and other applications are created outside of Blackboard and added into Blackboard courses for students to enhance teaching and learning efforts. TLC staffs also prepare class schedules for students enrolled in the programmes.

However, in order to better contribute to the goal of educating health professionals for the practice of community health/PHC, teaching and learning centres must have a community health-centric mission that incorporates the idea of lifelong learning aimed at improving the lives of communities who must be the primary beneficiaries. Thus, TLCs with such a mission can have many functions such as information centres, community centres, research centres and non-formal education activity centres to promote and provide lifelong learning based on the real needs of community health. As we have seen in Part One, Chapter 4 one of the much stressed important aspects of education in health care and learning in community is the development of a lifelong learner - an education which is seen as building upon and affecting all existing educational providers, including both schools and institutions of higher education, an education that extends beyond the formal educational providers to include all agencies, groups and individuals involved in any kind of learning activity, and an education that is grounded on the belief that individuals are, or can become, self-directing, and that they will see the value in engaging in lifelong education. We have also seen in Part One, Chapter 1, that a renewed primary health care system would have the characteristics of a more community-based primary health care organisations which focus on the specific needs of the individuals and populations they serve; greater coordination and integration with other health services, for example, hospitals and home care services; a greater emphasis on health promotion, illness and injury prevention and the management of chronic diseases, to help people to stay healthy and not just focus on treatment once they are sick; care provided by a team of primary health care providers (for example, nurses, family physicians, nutritionists, counsellors, just to name a few) so that the most appropriate care is provided by the most appropriate provider; and greater access to health services, so that people can get advice and care outside of regular office hours.

Teaching and learning centres can help to achieve all these by functioning as academic settings where (1) health professionals collaborate to develop comprehensive plans of care which will require professionals to take the time to get to know the skills that different professional groups bring to the primary health care setting; (2) primary health care teams include various frameworks through which to see clients and develop an understanding of, and responsive to, the changing needs of the communities they serve; and (3) health professionals take into account the physical, social and economic factors that impact upon individuals and shift the focus away from treating illness to broader social health focus. These are roles and functions that can be carried out by TLCs at each level of health care for primary health care teams and other agencies.

It is good practice to include a separate purpose for project management. Here, key project management tasks can be included as outputs such as staff management, financial management, and equipment maintenance. Such issues are further discussed in the final section on project governance.

**Outputs**

For each purpose, the community health education leader and his/her team should identify what outputs are necessary for the purpose to be achieved. They must make the outputs fit the real needs and avoid outputs that are not absolutely necessary. As any purpose can be achieved in several ways, they need to think creatively and analyse the advantages and disadvantages of different options before making a choice. The outputs that are necessary for the project purpose to be realised are, for example:

- increasing the number of health professional graduates opting for community health/PHC careers, as well as adding to the number of health professionals who are better educated and dedicated to the practice of PHC in

community health settings have been realised.
- use of the ICT-supported cooperative and collaborative learning modes that can engage students in many activities to form the social interactions needed to establish and build a community of learning for community health.

These outputs of the community health/PHC-centric teaching and learning centres focus on cooperative and collaborative teaching and learning through which community health educators and their partners can develop a dynamic and collaborative partnership between community health schools in university/colleges and community health service user, practice and policy communities. Through this partnership they will enhance and expand the delivery and evaluation of innovative interdisciplinary community health programmes within higher education and the community health sector. Service users' involvement as well as e-learning will be key features of programme development and evaluation. The centres will actively contribute to the promotion of best practice in supporting students to access and complete programmes of academic study.

### Activities

Each output is delivered via a set of activities. At the initial project design stage, the best way of achieving purposes and outputs may be unclear, so activities may need future finalisation and probably revision. Activities of teaching and learning centres, like their purposes and outputs, can be many and varied among institutions. However, there are typical activities that are carried out in these centres that are needed in community health education, including professional development services designed to help professionals improve their teaching and professional careers which TLCs typically offer. Examples of such faculty support services are outlined as follows:

## Faculty Support Services

- promote more modern teaching methods, discussions, and institutional changes in teaching practices and in the academic environment.
- sponsor and facilitate faculty learning communities (FLCs) for professional development in teaching. FLCs consist of instructors, often similar or related fields, to meet in small groups to troubleshoot difficulties and issues that they face in teaching, and to brainstorm or research solutions. Members meet regularly to discuss issues and findings, and may engage in journaling or other means of promoting reflective practice about their teaching. FLCs also promote a sense of community and sharing of teaching experience.
- offer workshops, meetings, or consultation services in other areas of professional development for teachers. This includes topics in teaching skills, such as improving one's lectures or course design for more student-centered and interesting lessons, teaching specific academic skills, using new instructional technologies, and help with presentation skills.
- address teacher-student issues that might include understanding and ad-

dressing difficulties that students might have; guidance on how to mentor graduate students; and understanding issues of gender, race or other factors that can affect classroom dynamics and academic performance.
- address evaluation and assessment issues like designing assignments, designing quizzes and exams, grading, and giving feedback.
- Provide career-related help for matters like help with writing grants, academic job search skills, and creating teaching portfolios for those seeking academic jobs.

Other Services
- provide support services for students in study and learning skills, or even peer tutoring programmes.
- provide support for e-learning and research on e-learning programmes and techniques.
- participate in e-learning movements and consortiums.
- conduct internal evaluations on the effectiveness of academic programmes, or may manage student feedback on instructors' performance.
- provide faculty help in understanding and making use of students' course feedback.
- conduct educational research on teaching methods or e-learning programmes.

Here again, the leader and his/her team must specify activities that teaching and learning centres should carry out that may include the above activities. However, activities specified must be consistent with the needs of community health education, including professional development services designed to help health professionals improve their teaching and professional careers and functioning in the complex community healthcare settings. Activities that can especially deliver the outputs of the project in the context of a renewed PHC are shown in Box 15:

Box 15: A Renewed PHC System: Five areas for Action
- build healthy public social policy
- create supportive environments
- strengthen community action
- re-orient health services
- develop individual personal skills

*Source: WHO (1987)*

These activities of TLCs should include mobilising community resources, encouraging community participation, and cooperating and networking with government and non-government organisations for promoting and providing lifelong learning activities; community needs assessment, planning and implementing the learning programmes and reporting, as well as fundraising activities which may be undertaken by local governments and social support groups for community health/PHC education development (e.g. UNESCO 2012).

The last action includes offering various educational programmes, such as workshops or meetings on various aspects of professional development and teaching techniques. Workshops may provide instruction in newer teaching techniques, by introducing techniques to instructors and/or helping them to better implement these methods. Newer or more student-centred techniques should include group activities, ICT-supported cooperative and collaborative learning, or non-traditional forms of assessment such as portfolios and formative assessment techniques. Faculty is prepared to facilitate cooperative and collaborative learning in community and prompt them to consider the value of 'community' in student learning. Orientation workshops can also introduce teaching skills as well as other necessary information for newer faculty members (e.g. CQ University 2011; UNESCO 2012).

Giving support services for students in study and learning skills, or even peer-tutoring programmes is a usual service that TLCs in community health often provide, but as indicated before, the activities of many TLCs that provide such services to students are still conditioned by the primary care model, which limits the role that such centres can play in community health/PHC education (Boaden et al 1999).

At this point it is important that the leader and his/her team test the above logic for checking and finalisation. Examples of logic testing questions are: (goal) does the goal indicate a higher-order impact or future intended state towards which the project is contributing? (Purpose) is the purpose a clear statement of what the project will realise generally? (Outputs) do all the outputs in total outline the group of achievements that must be realised for the outcomes to be realised? (Activities) do the activities that are carried out to achieve each output produce the main actions that must occur for the outputs to be achieved? Finally, the leader and his/her team must question, for instance, whether project stakeholders comprehend all levels of the logic as clearly as possible (IFAD 2011).

**Resources**

The leader and his/her team must allocate resources required for activities and develop an overall budget. In addition to making specific demands on the expertise and skills of teachers, community-based curriculum development, implementation and evaluation will also raise questions on resources limitations. Such undertakings demand energy and finance, not to mention, among other things, the time of community health educators have to deal with, such as the problem of work overload and lack of facilities and materials in TLCs located especially in developing countries. The team leader and teachers should analyse the financial, technical and managerial aspects of TLC policy with a view to assessing the accessibility of resources, and to judging how resources can be assembled to guarantee increased practical implementation of TLC policy. The key is to assemble such resources to strengthen policy reforms. This is because people, who are not resistant to change, may subsequently encounter difficulties that will constrain their efforts to implement change (Gross 1971). It is clear from the above discussion that sufficient or appropriately channelled financial resources from the three tiers of PHC-tertiary, secondary and primary levels, and managerial resources, such as appropriate infrastructure, adequate technical support, capable human resources, resource materials and space for discussions are crucial factors when implementing professional development programmes in TLCs. In fact, efforts aimed at implementing education policy reforms have shown that changes in policy were most often reported from countries with high economic development (Sobral et al 1978).

As we have seen in Part One, Chapter 6, according to the Resource Dependence theory (Pfeffer et al 1978), the primary motivator for organisational behaviour is the desire to reduce uncertainty about getting the resources necessary to operate. These resources include financial, key personnel, seats on influential community boards, or contacts with prestigious organisations, space, budgets, equipment, and community agencies and groups. To be effective, community health faculty leaders must be able to accurately analyse power issues both within an agency and within the community. They must be able to predict the resource requirements of the agency and how managing those resources may affect power issues within the system (Pfeffer et al 1978). Faculty leaders must try to ensure that they have adequate resources to achieve their mission, vision, and goals for the building of community of learning intervention.

Therefore, governments and community health managers of TLCs in especially poor countries should explore the possibility of securing support from funding mechanisms that can greatly enhance relevant continuing education policy implementation, such as the one used by the WHO (Jancloes 1998) to develop an intensified approach for cooperation with countries and people in greatest need in order to improve the implementation of primary health care. This approach includes preliminary missions to countries, consultations with international agencies and joint missions with multilateral and bilateral cooperating agencies, material and technical assistance through WHO Regional Offices, and earmarking of funds to enable WHO technical programmes to focus attention on selected countries.

There are other ways through which communities in poor countries are able to mobilise support for community health and TLCs, such as community financing mechanisms that are managed by communities themselves. This case study account (Eklund et al 1990) about a health insurance financing scheme in Guinea-Bissau, West Africa, provides a good example of the kinds of insurance schemes that can be adopted for financing the TLC development project at the community level. A community insurance scheme was established in this country to pay for drugs at village level, which were dispensed by the Village Health Worker. Adopted by a few villages when it began in 1980, the scheme grew ten years later to become a national programme catering for more than twenty-percent of the population. The major reason for implementing this prepayment scheme, as opposed to user fees, is its administrative plainness.

After harvest each year a village leader would simply visit each household to ask for payment of a fixed amount. The community was responsible for deciding the amount and collecting the money to finance the continued supply of drugs. Those who paid the annual insurance contribution were given a receipt, entitling the holders, including women and their children, to free drugs and consultations. The scheme received a significant leap in 1983 from the ministry of health when it agreed to accept members of the scheme referred by Village Health Workers (VHWs) to government health facilities without members paying the fee that they normally would have paid before receiving care. Although increasing economic pressure finally led to misuse of funds that threatened the credibility of the scheme, the villages managed the scheme well.

But it must be emphasised that the burdens of funding PHC and professional development programmes that are provided within community health/PHC systems should not fall mostly on the poor. Because developing countries are particularly poor and resources have fallen far below what is considered necessary to provide effective health services, most of these policy reforms would require major financial injections into the national health budget. Even where this is possible through international aid or national means, it will not guarantee positive outcomes in resource use in the absence of social capital. As outlined in Part One, Chapter 7, social capital refers to the components of social life, namely, the existence of networks, policies, institutions, relationships and norms.

As discussed, these aspects of social life enable people to act together, create synergies and build partnerships. In order to preserve social capital for sustained economic growth and development it is necessary to foster networks of trust and knowledge creation and sharing at the organisational, community and regional as well as between different sectors such as government, higher education and business (OECD 2005). Social capital also requires the maintenance and replenishment of shared values by communities, social and religious groups (Goodland et al 1996). Studies (Lisagor 2013) have found that communities with strong social capital are more likely to bounce back than those with fewer social resources. It also means that service projects must involve intensive discussions between donors and recipients, as well as fellowship that fosters the building of social capital and, therefore, effective use of resources.

**Work schedule**

The leader and his/her team must develop a work schedule for the main activities over the life of the project and establish key milestones. The purpose of the schedule is to define timelines for key deliverables and sets expectations for project progress and completion. The leader uses the schedule to help plan, execute and control project tasks and to track and monitor the progress of the project. The project schedule describes time (duration) estimates for all project tasks, start and finish dates for the tasks, names of staff, resources assigned to complete the tasks, and sequence of tasks. The project schedule is constructed to reflect the work breakdown structure, which is a major component of a project schedule. The project schedule information is included in the project plan (e.g. Microsoft Corporation 2014).

Be it as it may, such a schedule must allow for certain critical tasks to be performed in the TLCs: development of comprehensive plans of care or programmes by health professionals, which will demand professionals to collaborate with each other and with other members of the multidisciplinary team; primary health care teams learning to include various frameworks through which to see clients or develop programmes, and in doing so develop an understanding of, and responsive to, the changing needs of the communities they serve, and considering the physical, social and economic factors that impact upon individuals and shift the focus away from treating illness to broader social health focus (Boaden et al 1999).

All these require work schedules in TLCs that, as we indicated earlier, are comprehensive enough and do not at times encourage a model of provision which is expensive, making TLCs not easily used by practitioners that require the services they provide. Such services, as we have seen, are often oriented around the institutional norms of higher education, involving formal qualifications and the structure of provision corresponding with the traditional demands of such qualifications. TLC facilities are also used by the minority of practitioners, or by those who have to wait for their turn, be given study leave and have the needed time for study. As was suggested, community-based practice needs a different approach that involves distance learning that allows practitioners to attend periodically local facilities to give the needed contact which is often not possible with formal courses, access to educational material organised in a way that facilities use, and short-term courses (Boaden et al 1999). The leader and his/her team must develop the kind of work schedules needed for accommodating such professional development activities and needs. This leads to consideration of the management and operational arrangements of TLCs in the community

## Management and operational arrangements

Establishing the management and operational arrangements with key responsibilities and working procedures is also another task of the leader and his/her team. As developing a good project strategy does not happen in one go from top to bottom, they will need to return to earlier steps as thinking becomes more detailed. For example, when you start thinking about the cost and practicality of some activities you realise that some outputs and purposes might be unrealistic. Therefore, the leader and his/her team need to establish a decision-making framework that is logical, robust and repeatable to govern a teaching and learning centre's capital investments. This way the centre will have a structured approach to conducting both its business as usual activities and its business change, or project activities (e.g Williams 2012; IFAD 2011).

This decision-making framework can be supported by the project governance pillars of structure, people and information (Williams 2012). Structure involves governance committee structure, for example, a project board or a project steering committee, ideally a broader governance environment that may include various stakeholder groups and perhaps user groups. In addition, there may be a programme board, governing a group of related projects of which this is one, and possibly some form of portfolio decision-making group. The decision rights of all these committees and how they relate must be laid down in policy and procedural documentation. In this way, the project's governance can be integrated within the wider governance arena.

It is people who populate the various governance committees that the governance structure rests upon. Committee membership is determined by the characteristics of the project, but other factors may be considered when deciding membership of programme and portfolio boards. This in turn determines which organisational roles should be tabled on the committee. Information is concerned with the information that informs decision makers and consists of regular reports on the project, issues and risks that have been escalated by the project manager and certain key documents that describe the project, the business case being the most important of these.

Figure 5 presents an example (University of British Colombia (UBC 2013) of how management and operational arrangements of teaching and learning centres can be established in a university. It shows the high-level organisational context of the Centre for Teaching, Learning and Technology of the university. The Centre reports to the Provost through the Vice Provost and Associate Vice President Academic Affairs. The Centre is co-led by an Academic Director and a Managing Director. The Academic Director also serves as Senior Advisor, Teaching and Learning. As the organisational chart indicates, the Senior Advisor role acts independently of the CTLT and facilitates interaction amongst the different teaching and learning enterprises of the university.

**Figure 5: UBC Vancouver Centre for Teaching, Learning and Technology Organisational Context and Operational Framework**

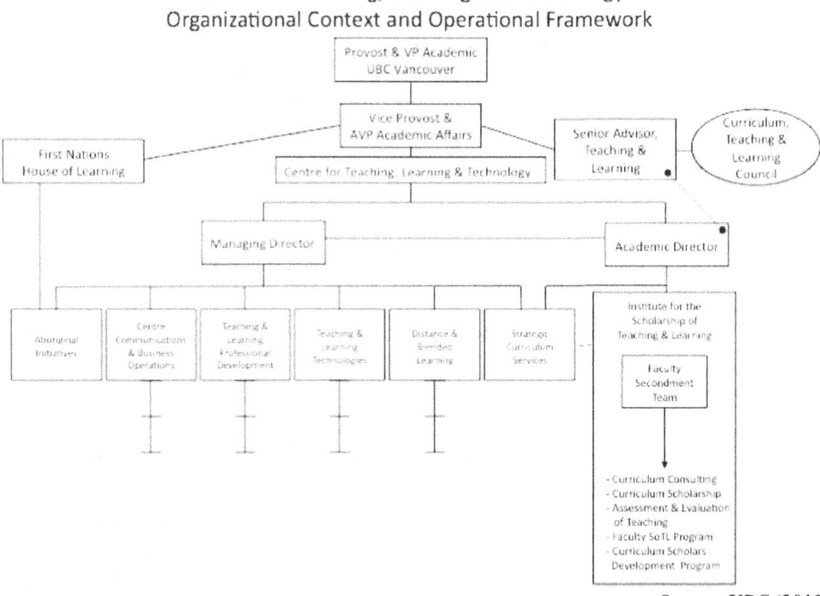


*Source: UBC (2013)*

This approach is said to highlight the benefits of strong leadership (academic and management) along with the need for integration of teaching, learning and technology. Furthermore, the Institute for the Scholarship of Teaching and Learning (ISOTL) is better resourced to advance scholarly approaches to curriculum and pedagogy within and across the disciplines, as well as support the scholarship of educational practice within these contexts. New opportunities within the Institute are planned to engage faculty members more deeply with CTLT as well strengthen and advance UBC's ability to provide an exceptional learning environment to its learning community.

There is evidence to suggest that this is a common organisational structure that reflects the management and operational arrangements with key responsibilities and working procedures in many university-based teaching and learning centres in developed countries even where their missions include health (e.g. Ukaigwe 2013; CQ University 2011)). In the example presented above (Ukaigwe 2013), in which the university teaching and learning centre manages educational programmes in a variety of disciplines including courses on global health there is an office for teaching and learning headed by a Provost and Vice President with similar management and operational arrangements.

As we have seen in Part One, Chapter 7, as organisations like universities grow larger they become more highly formalised or structured. The real reason for establishing governance structures within a project is the recognition that organisation structures like the one Figure 1 shows do not provide the necessary framework to deliver a project. Unlike organisation charts that are linked to hierarchical mechanisms that the figure demonstrates, project governance structures overcome this by drawing the key decision makers out of the organisation structure and putting them in a forum thereby avoiding the serial decision-making process associated with hierarchies. As a result, the project governance framework established for a project should remain separate from the organisation structure.

Adoption of this principle will minimise multi-layered decision-making and the time delays and inefficiencies associated with it. It will ensure a project decision-making body empowered to make decisions in a timely manner. Thus, in decentralised systems of continuing education/professional development (UNESCO 2012) the management of Community Learning Centres, for instance, can be left in the hands of teachers/facilitators and CLC committees, groups of CLCs management and teaching, who may be permanent staff, part-time staff or community volunteers. We will discuss this approach to decentralisation of continuing education later in this chapter.

The recognition of this principle and approaches used to put it into practice are demonstrated by examples of how countries in the developing world that have adopted the PHC approach have decentralised continuing education delivery including in the community. A decentralised organisation is one in which decision-making is not confined to a few top executives but rather is done throughout the organisation, with managers at various levels making key operating decisions relating to their sphere of responsibility. Decentralisation is a matter of degree, since all organisations are decentralised to some extent out of necessity. At one extreme, a strongly decentralised organisation is one in which even the lowest-level managers and employees are empowered to make decisions. At the other extreme, in a strongly centralised organisation, lower-level managers have little freedom to make decisions. Although most organisations fall somewhere between these two extremes, there is a pronounced trend towards more and more decentralisation (Collins et al 1994).

In education, most governments have experienced the deficiencies of centralised education service provision, which include especially administrative and fiscal inefficiency, opaque decision-making, and poor quality and access to services and, therefore, the theoretical advantages of decentralisation have become extremely appealing. Generally, the decentralisation process can significantly improve transparency, efficiency, responsiveness of service provision and accountability when compared with centralised systems. Decentralising the provision of education provision pledges to better reflect local priorities, be more efficient, enhances participation, and, eventually, improves coverage and quality. Especially countries experiencing severe fiscal constraints are enticed by the potential of decentralisation to increase efficiency. Cost recovery schemes such as community financing in many communities have been established to help fund education service provision that had been funded entirely by governments (World Bank Group 2001).

The general argument for decentralising health care is the potential for improved service quality and coverage. Health care decentralisation is a highly popular concept, being a key element of Primary Health Care policies. This is reflected by the delivery of health services in the many developing countries that have adopted the PHC approach which is through a three-tier system of tertiary, intermediate and primary levels. For example, the Gambian PHC structure is comprised of:

- The village is the basic unit for the delivery of Primary Health Care. Here Traditional Birth Attendants (TBAs) and Village Health Workers (VHWs) provide the village health services. They are supervised by Community Health Nurses who are stationed at PHC key villages.

- Health centres (major and minor) and Dispensaries at the intermediate (or secondary) level serve as the base from which mobile health services are organised to provide services to underserved areas.

- The tertiary level consists mainly of urban health services. There are several hospitals that are located in various parts of the country, mainly in the urban and peri-urban areas. There are many private clinics and numerous private physicians and pharmacies.

At all these three levels there are many non-governmental organisations providing both preventative and curative services in the rural and urban settings.

There are roles and functions at each level of such a three-tier system for ministries of health and other stakeholders in the management and operations of professional development in the countries. For example (Adefunmike 2013), there are at the Federal Government level (tertiary level) in one teaching hospital a Teaching Hospital Governing Board under which operates a General Administration section and a Clinical Services Department. The General Administration section directs the affairs of a Residency and Training Programmes Department which approves training and development programmes, regularises training and recommends release of health professionals for training and development with or without sponsorship. The Clinical Services Department is responsible for training and development of health professionals in a specific discipline which is normally conducted in training units specific to that discipline. For instance, there is a Community Medicine & Primary Healthcare Training Unit that is responsible for the training and development of physicians in relation to PHC/Community health. This unit is jointly owned by the university and the teaching hospital.

At the local government level (the village) managers are in direct contact with the community with regard to training and professional development. They are responsible for training and developing health professionals in relation to the eight principal elements of PHC (Part One, Chapter 1), such as prevention and control of locally endemic diseases. Here also a training and development unit is established for each discipline, for instance, nursing. The Director of Primary Health Care coordinates such training and through him/her health professionals are placed in different units for training. Although there may be differences between countries, basically a somewhat similar governance structure for health professional training and development exists in many developing countries whose health systems are based on the PHC approach.

However, a common governance structure considered an especially important means for decentralisation of service delivery as well as training and development is the health team's structure that is based in health divisions, regions, etc., at the intermediate levels of PHC. As already mentioned, the objectives of practice in the community should concentrate on, among other things, primary prevention and therapeutic care aimed at improving patient, family, and community health, and self-care. All these happen within a health delivery system that is based on the premise of primary health care for all; involving other sectors that influence health, using the health team approach. Box 16 shows the composition of one Regional Health Team

**Box 16: A Renewed PHC System: Five areas for Action**

- Director
- Principal Nursing Officer
- Principal Public Health Officer
- Senior Administrator
- Senior Community Health Nurse Tutor
- National Nutrition Agency Focal Person
- TB/Leprosy Focal Person
- Vector Control Officer
- Health Education Officer

*Source: Sabally (2013)*

All members of the team work with the Director and Senior Administrator (responsible for purchasing, maintenance, resources, etc) in managing the training and development of health personnel. Members of the team together with staff in the health facilities (e.g. health centres and dispensaries) at this level are responsible for training and development of health personnel. Any member of the team can also participate in the implementation of such training and development, particularly if the focus of the training and development is on his/her area of responsibility, for instance, vector control.

At the community level the Senior Community Health Nurse Tutor and community health nurses working in the community are responsible for training and development activities. Here again any DHT member can also participate in the implementation of such training and development activities at this level. Some of these activities at this level are carried out in community clinics established by communities. In these day-clinics services such as out-patient, health education, preventive and promotional, family planning, maternal and child health and outreach services are provided. These community clinics can therefore serve as learning centres where training and development can be better provided to community health personnel. Clinics and health centres are settings in which doctors, nurses, midwives, students, etc., collaborate. These healthcare arenas can, for example, help to coordinate activities between biomedical and ethno-medical practitioners who provide basic health services in many villages and form the nucleus of primary health workers in the majority of our local populations. Such integrated clinics which can become centres for research on medical plants, for instance, should provide a culturally holistic approach to illness and student learning in various aspects of primary health care and community health including appropriate technology, traditional medicine, etc.

In Chapter 8 we outlined several tips for undertaking new capital learning space design projects in the community, pointing out how these tips can be applied in building a community of learning in community, including designing capital learning space projects in teaching and learning centres at the local level of health care that have a community health-centric mission. Such a construction project, as we have seen, produces a complex system with human and mechanical components and the value generated by the project is embedded in the system. Such a project is also meant to produce an operationally effective process in teaching and learning centres. All that has been said about learning space design in Part Two, Chapter 1 applies to designing learning space in healthcare environments like the health centre and community health clinic, including the suggested pedagogical and curricular approaches, as well as the implications for designing learning environments to foster a community of learning. It also includes factors that can influence learning environment design in community health education, namely, levels or scope of health service delivery, type of organisation, style of management, professional staff in the settings, and the type of clients and their access to services.

For one to better understand the tips outlined in that and further discussion in relation to TLCs and to provide an example on which to situate the points that will be made here, it is helpful for one to consider the nature of the community health centre. A health centre or community health centre is a clinic staffed by a group of general practitioners and nurses. Typically, the services provided are family practice and dental care. However, some health centres implement a model for offering free services to certain population groups, such as rapid HIV testing to all patients between the ages of 13 and 64 during routine primary medical and dental care visits (Agency for Health Research and Quality 2013).

In developed countries like the USA, community health centres (CHCs) are neighbourhood health centres generally serving areas that are underserved, including areas where persons are uninsured, underinsured, low-income or those living in areas where little access to primary health care is available (Web 2012). These CHCs are mainly federally and locally funded. In such a developed country, some health clinics are modernised with new equipment and electronic medical records (Web 2012).

Table 40 shows the kind of comprehensive health services that are delivered in health systems of many developing countries that have adopted the PHC approach. As we indicated above, it is in settings like community health clinics or centres (referred to in Table 40 as minor health centre) and major health centres where whole health services may be delivered. Obviously, such settings can provide the professional development needs of community health professionals for better preparation in PHC, as well as needs for more skills in PHC in the community and in healthcare clinics, and in work in different sectors of health care systems.

Community health educators and their collaborators need to look at what learning space is needed in such healthcare settings, and how the learning environment can be designed and used in especially settings like the health centre. As we have seen, the health centres and clinics are serving as arenas for, among other things, the delivery of professional development/ continuing education in both developed and developing countries, especially developing countries (Adefunmike 2013).

However, the educational benefits that can result from integrating the education of health professionals with such health and social systems which can indeed be significant may be difficult to achieve due to many factors, including managers at community clinics not being empowered to make decisions. In this example, as in other examples from many countries where community clinics exist, decentralisation is a highly popular concept as, mentioned earlier, it is a principal requirement of Primary Health Care. But at the level of the community, planning of training and development programmes are usually carried out at the level of the DHT led by agencies funding these programmes without the participation of staff working at the local level in the planning. As we have seen, decentralisation is a matter of degree, since all organisations are decentralised to some extent out of necessity. The process transfers decision-making powers from central ministries of health to intermediate governments, local governments and communities. The extent of the transfer varies, however, from administrative decentralisation to much broader transfer of financial control to the regional or local level.

We have seen in Part One, Chapter 6, that community health leaders should work with community members to identify community health needs and policies

**Table 40: Healthcare Delivery in The Gambia**

| VHS | Minor H/C | Major H/C | Regional Hospital | Teaching Hospital |
|---|---|---|---|---|
| • Primary care service (including treatment of minor illnesses and referrals, environmental health & sanitation, antenatal, delivery and postpartum care, home visits, community health promotion activities s | • Maternity care (antenatal, delivery and postpartum<br>• Family Planning<br>• STIs prevention and control<br>• Immunisation<br>• Neonatal and child health<br>• Maternal and child nutrition<br>• Basic emergency maternal and obstetric care<br>• Disease prevention and control ( malaria, TB, etc)<br>• Health protection and control<br>• Basic Lab services(HB, BF, VDRL, Urine analysis TB and HIV screening)<br>• in-patient service<br>• Referral services<br>• Dispensary<br>• Eye care services<br>• Out-patient services<br>• Registration of births and Deaths | • All services provided at minor H/C level<br>• Comprehensive emergency obstetric care (including theatre and blood transfusion services)<br>• Functional theatre<br>• Comprehensive emergency newborn care<br>• In-patient services<br>• Pharmacy Services<br>• Basic Lab. services including HIV and TB Screening. | • All services provided at major H/C level<br>• Specialist care and service<br>• Higher level referral services<br>• Specialised dental and eye care services<br>• Comprehensive laboratory services<br>• Radiology services | • All services provided at regional hospital level<br>• Specialist hospital services (in- and out-patient services)<br>• Post-mortem and embalmment services<br>• Overseas referral |

*Source: MOH&SW (2012)*

and programmes (Orlando 1990); that even within large organisations individual units often function independently, giving a great deal of authority and responsibilities to managers, which empowers them to work in environments that support autonomy (Burns 1978). However, in other cases organisational leaders choose a more centralised approach, in part because these structures tend to be less costly and wasteful, especially in resource constraint healthcare settings (Pfeffer 1982). This may be why despite the strong drive for decentralisation of health and education programmes in developing countries often little has been achieved in efforts at such decentralisation. As already indicated, loose or organically structured organisation, are more likely to be decentralised, with much decision-making authority pushed down to the lowest level in the agency where employees have the information needed for making decisions.

Moreover, not only can large committees that may be produced by decentralisation processes in the community fail to make timely decisions, those that do are often ill considered because of the particular group dynamics at play. A number of roadblocks limit community learning. Different communication styles and values in higher education subcultures such as students, facilities managers, faculty, etc, can block collaboration. Differences in knowledge and expertise, personality differences and group dynamics can also present roadblocks. Additionally, roadblocks can emanate from processes and systems that can prevent people from reaching a consensus (Bickford et al 2010). For example, it is challenging to manage a multi-owned TLC for several reasons, such as putting a mechanism in place to summon independent review or scrutiny when it is in the legitimate interests of one or more of the project owners. This is why large project committees are constituted more as a stakeholder management forum than a project decision-making forum. This is a major issue when the project is depending upon the committee to make timely decisions.

As project decision-making forums grow in size, they tend to develop into stakeholder management groups. When numbers increase, the detailed understanding of each attendee of the critical project issues reduces. Many of those present attend not to make decisions but to find out what is happening on the project. Not only is there insufficient time for each person to make their point, but those with the most valid input must compete for time and influence with those with only a peripheral involvement in the project. Furthermore, not all present will have the same level of understanding of the issues and so time is wasted bringing everyone up to speed on the particular issues being discussed. Hence, to all intents and purposes, large project committees are constituted more as a stakeholder management forum than a project decision-making forum. This is a major issue when the project is depending upon the committee to make timely decisions. However, it must be realised that both activities - project decision making and stakeholder management - are essential to the success of the project.

Apart from the difficulty of empowering staff at the local level to make decisions, there is the issue of who in the organisation should be held accountable. The concept of a single point of accountability is the first principle of effective project governance. The person nominated must be the right person to be made accountable. However, this person must hold sufficient authority within the organisation and to ensure that he/she is empowered to make the decisions necessary for the project's success. Many teaching and learning centres in community health education may be based in universities and colleges from where a leader leads a team of community health educators to teach at teaching and learning centres or continuing education units (e.g. Adefunmike 2013) located in the community. As has been mentioned, for a leader to be able to tap into the potential of community, he or she must possess certain qualities, and in addition the leader must be empowered to carry out the needed tasks. The leader must focus on the best ways to organise work, on how to obtain the resources necessary to accomplish agency goals, on organisational level change, and on power dynamics, as well as be able to deal with the dynamics of rapid, interconnected change and the emergence of patterns of activity in teaching and learning centres.

There is the issue of who plays the project owner role. Usually, organisations promote the allocation of the project owner role to the service owner or asset owner with the goal of providing more certainty that the project will meet these owner's fundamental needs, which is also a critical project success measure. This may be the case in community settings where professional development programmes are delivered. However, the result of this approach can involve wasteful inclusions and failure to achieve alternative stakeholder and customer requirements, such as project owner requirements receiving less scrutiny, reducing innovation and reducing outcome efficiency.

Community health managers need to consider what policy to follow where teaching and learning centre projects are multi-owned. A multi-owned project is one in which the board shares ultimate control with other parties. Ownership of TLCs may be by governments or ministries of health, but also by community organisations and foundations. As already mentioned, there are Academic Primary Health Care centres owned jointly and operated under partnerships based in the community. Continuing education units may also be jointly owned by universities/colleges and teaching hospitals. Managers can take the following course of action where TLCs are jointly-owned (Department of Education and Early Childhood Development 2007):

- Formally agreeing with partners' governance arrangements.
- Agreeing with partners on a single point of decision- making for the project.
- Making clear the person who has authority for representing the project in contacts with owners, stakeholders and third parties.
- Including in the project business case agreed, and current, definitions of project objectives, the role of each owner, their incentives, inputs, authority and responsibility.
- Making the legal competence and obligations and internal governance arrangements of each co-owner compatible with its acceptable standards of governance for the project.
- Giving owners the necessary degree of control over the project through project authorisation points and limiting constraints.
- Agreeing on recognition and allocation or sharing of rewards and risks taking

into account ability to influence the outcome and creating incentives to foster cooperative behaviour.

- Exploiting synergies arising from multi-ownership and actively managing potential sources of conflict or inefficiency.
- Formally agreeing on the definition of the process to be cited and the consequences for assets and owners when a material change of ownership is considered.
- Providing honest, timely, realistic and relevant data on progress, achievements, forecasts and risks to the extent required for good governance by owners when reporting during both the project and the realisation of benefits.
- Putting a mechanism in place to summon independent review or scrutiny when it is in the legitimate interests of one or more of the project owners.
- Agreeing with other owners a dispute resolution process that does not endanger the achievement of project objectives.

There are lessons to be learned from experiences of several countries concerning decentralisation and planning of the delivery of continuing education through Community Learning Centres in many countries. For instance, there are efforts by countries of the Asia-Pacific region to decentralise continuing education delivery including at the community level contained in a report on the Asia-Pacific Regional Conference on Community learning centres (UNESCO 2012). In these countries the Community Learning Centre (CLC) Project was launched in 1998 in the framework of the UNESCO Asia-Pacific Programme of Education for All (APPEAL). The purpose of CLCs is to promote human development by providing opportunities for lifelong learning to all people in local communities. CLCs support empowerment, social transformation and improvement of the quality of life (UNESCO 2012).

The main functions of CLCs are to provide: (a) education and training (b) community information and resource services (c) community development activities, and (d) coordination and networking. The presence of CLCs in some countries in the region has greatly expanded. CLCs have been largely serving people at the grassroots level in more than 20 countries in Asia and Pacific. However, it has been difficult to keep all CLCs functioning at a high standard. Rapid expansion of the number of CLCs has sacrificed the quality of their programme delivery in some countries. Inadequate technical support, poor infrastructure, lack of resource materials, lack of space for discussions, and lack of capable human resources are the main reasons for low performance. Development of a set of standards and a system for quality assurance are considered necessary to improve the quality of the programmes in these countries.

Decentralisation of the delivery mechanism of continuing education and management of CLCs, which is one of the key issues on which the conference exchanged experiences and ideas, has been promoted and countries face difficulties to put it into practice effectively due mainly to the problems outlined above. The report suggests the following measures for tackling difficulties on decentralisation and the related issue of literacy policy and planning which the conference also considered:

**Decentralisation**

- Clear government structure and roles of government from the local to national levels, which support transparency and accountability.
- Enabling policies and regulations as the prerequisite for establishing an effective mechanism of programme delivery.
- Continuous capacity development at all levels to make the mechanism work effectively.
- Strengthening of capacity and ownership with strong local leadership is essential.

**Policy and Planning**

- Legislation for non-formal education as well as national plans plays an important role for scaling up and speeding up the attainment of the literacy goal.
- More evidence-based analysis, consultations and discussions are needed for formulation of legislation and plans.
- Prioritisation is critical to make policies and plans more realistic and feasible to implement rather than just creating a long list of activities.
- Well co-ordinated UN agencies and donor groups with sound policy documents are necessary for convincing government authorities and ensuring a reasonable budget.
- Literacy needs to be linked to other sectors to ensure fund mobility.
- Credible data and information are essential for formulation of policy and planning
- Expanding post-literacy programmes is also necessary (UNESCO 2012).

Clearly the characteristics, purposes and activities of the CLCs in decentralised system of continuing education, as well as many of the conclusions on CLCs made by the conference reflect significantly the concepts of learning, the principles of PHC/community health and the good practices of designing any development intervention we outlined in Part One. For instance, as mentioned there, one of the much stressed important aspects of education in health care and learning in community is the development of a lifelong learner. The difficulties faced in the management of CLCs are also not that different from the constraints community health managers of professional development programmes and TLCs have to deal with in especially many developing countries where programme delivery has been decentralised in the context of PHC, such as lack of funding and inadequate facilities. The proposals for tackling the problems of managing CLCs in decentralised systems much of which have been covered in the previous chapter on the needed changes in education and healthcare systems to support professional development/continuing education are equally important for community health managers to consider. For example, they must realise that decentralisation must include strengthening lower level management capacity in PHC systems. Managers must know that decentralisation cannot successfully provide PHC if the local government is restricted to operate by being vulnerable to, for instance, locally dominant groups. While there must be some degree of centralisation in resource allocation and planning for PHC, the proposed form of decentralisation should promote and not hinder policies of equity. For example, as already mentioned, the burdens of funding PHC and professional development that is provided within PHC systems should not fall mostly on the poor. Managers and policymakers must consider whether the proposed form of decentralisation will or will not provide more for those in the greatest need (Collins et al 1994).

The Asian Pacific Regional Conference on Community Learning Centres also deliberated on five key issues facing CLCs other than decentralisation and policy and planning to increase knowledge for effective operation and implementation of CLC/continuing education programmes. The other five key issues are:

- Quality assurance of CLCs
- Regional exchange and platform of CLCs
- Learning content for the twenty-first century (Equivalency Programmes and Education for Sustainable Development)
- ICT and continuing education
- Literacy assessment and monitoring programmes for monitoring literacy skills levels of the population in host countries

Findings from the conference on these key issues are concluded as follows:

**Quality Assurance: Monitoring and Evaluation**

- There is need to assess multiple aspects of CLC programmes, the purpose of which should be clear to ensure concrete follow-up actions.
- Assessment must focus on both quality and quantity.
- Assessment needs to be conducted and participated in, by internal and external evaluators, as well as by people in the community who manage and benefit from CLC activities.
- Creating a quality assurance system with clear standards which can regularly monitor and evaluate the programmes of CLCs in terms of their delivery and achievements.

**Innovation for Sustaining Community-based Literacy and Continuing Education Delivery Mechanisms**

- Learning needs to be rooted in the cultural context.
- Important factors to sustain CLCs are diversified learning curricula which relate to improved living conditions and the clear roles of stakeholders in CLCs.
- Establishing synergy of community ownership and external support are also crucial for ensuring the sustainability of CLCs.
- It is crucial to ensure "readiness" of a community prior to opening a CLC.
- It is important to build both the capacities of community and of external supporters to understand the local context and mechanisms for success and to decide how best to provide external assistance.

**Emerging Learning Content for twenty-first Century Delivery to CLCs**

- Learning is at the core of coping with change.
- Learning needs are diversified in a world of constant change and flux.
- Information and communication technologies (ICTs) have the potential to work as an engine for change and to create networks.
- Connecting people and encouraging collaboration among people will be an effective approach to emerging learning content.
- Approaches that combine new technologies such as ICT, traditional media such as newspapers and community radio should be sustained.
- Concentration of knowledge and skills continues to take place and we face increasing polarisation which represents a socio-economic divide.
- Continuous professional development is more important than ever.
- Learning needs should be constantly reviewed.
- Whatever the approaches and content of learning are, it is important to recognise that human beings and sustainability are at the centre of learning for a harmonisation of environmental well-being, economic viability and a more just society.
- In addition to the four pillars of learning, learning to know, learning to do, learning to be, and learning to live together, which UNESCO promotes, the fifth pillar, "learning to transform," shall be added to build a sustainable future.

**Effective Application of ICT in Literacy and Continuing Education**

- Learning can be more effective through the use of ICT.
- It is important to recognise and advocate that ICT is not a replacement of the traditional tools for learning, but rather a supplement to enhance learning.
- In order to efficiently use ICT in education and learning, capacity development at all levels is necessary, especially for teachers and facilitators.
- ICT devices proved to be effective to attract and connect learners.
- Traditional ICT tools like television and radio are still useful for education and learning.
- To address equity issues it is crucial to narrow the digital divide.

**Global Initiatives and Regional Networks**

- The national reports will be synthesised and published as "Global Report on Adult Learning and Education".
- The reporting process shall be used to further enhance advocacy and capacity building in the field of adult education in target countries.
- In addition to international, regional and national networks, sub regional co-operation needs to be enhanced to promote exchange and sharing of ideas, experiences and resources.
- The idea and potential of an International CLC Association at regional and sub regional levels were well appreciated.
- However, more discussion will be required on its standards and policies of membership, an accepted definition of CLC, and its function among stake-

holders.

- Due to the rapid advancement and affordability of ICT, connecting CLCs across countries has become easier through social networks like Facebook.
- Mutual learning and information sharing can be promoted more widely among CLCs. LIFE portals are being created for nine LIFE countries in the Asia-Pacific region.
- They will function as a platform to collect documents and materials for knowledge sharing, as a discussion forum in LIFE countries and to help accelerate programmes to meet the literacy goals.

It is apparent that the conclusions/suggestions on these other five key critical issues facing CLCs are reflective of or are in agreement with many of the theories, concepts, principles and approaches we outlined in chapters in Part One on community health/ a renewed PHC, education, curricula, learning, particularly the ideas of learning in community and building community of learning, technology, communication and information exchange, ICT and learning, leadership and management, as well as the good practices of designing any development intervention, which incorporates the important concepts of self-reliance and sustainability. The conclusions/suggestions are also consistent with points made in subsequent chapters on technology, community and information, and curricular and co-curricular design. Perhaps particularly interesting of all the conclusions are suggestions under learning content for 21st delivery of CLCs, effective ICT application in literacy and continuing education and innovations for sustaining community-based literacy and continuing education delivery mechanisms.

These suggestions corroborate the major thesis of this book: how to build a community of learning in community health education in the 21st century. As mentioned earlier, faculty, students and communities can engage and learn from each other to re-build community and enhance learning in community through three strategic community processes (Bickford et al (2010): (1) designing learning spaces (2) using information, communication technology, and (3) designing pedagogy, curricula and co-curricular activities for learning. These three strategic community processes can interact to build community that fosters learning in community health. They include good practices in any design process of any development intervention (IFAD 2011) that reflect the PHC principles of self-reliance, equity, community participation and inter-sectoral collaboration - the ideas that are integrated into the practice of community health care in homes, dispensaries, health centres and hospitals, which constitute the different levels of health care (WHO 1986).

In discussing the important issue of identifying professional development needs for community health in the previous chapter, we started by making two points. One is that professional development in community health does not only consist of traditional training which is required to cover essential work-related skills, techniques and knowledge, but most importantly it also enables learning and personal development, which the above suggestions/conclusions also reflect. We mentioned that learning and personal development extend the range of development way outside conventional work skills and knowledge, and creates far more exciting, liberating, motivational opportunities for people and for employers. We also mentioned that healthcare systems are increasingly being more complex and changing rapidly.

Consequently, organisations in health care are facing great pressure to change nowadays in order to facilitate and encourage development and fulfilment of the whole person additionally to traditional training. The second point we made is that community health educators should use curriculum planning models and approaches (Part One, Chapter 3) that can adequately accommodate the realities that account for the limitations in PHC and community-oriented education and practice. Both intentions are required for sustaining community-based learning and effective change in community health systems and must constitute major learning content in community health education, including community of learning in the 21st century. We have also stressed the importance of ICT-supported cooperative and collaborative learning in fostering community of learning in community health. These two modes of learning are considered the most important learning strategy for succeeding with the aim of designing learning processes that are needed for building community of learning,

On the issue of effective application of ICT in continuing education/professional development in the community, the suggestion from the conference that traditional media like television and radio are still useful for education reflects existing practices in the use of ICT in PHC/community health education contexts especially in developing countries. As already mentioned, broadcast technologies such as radio and television have a much greater penetration than the Internet throughout much of the developing world, and that this substantial gap is not expected to be closed soon, due to cost, etc. These ICTs are therefore consistent with the concept of appropriate technology which we highlighted in previous chapters. As we have seen in these and previous chapters there are increasing efforts to utilise other ICT applications like telemedicine in healthcare education settings. But we need to consider especially the application of such an ICT in settings such as the health centre and clinics where community health education can be more targeted to the needs of specific communities.

For instance, let us take the setting up of a telemedicine unit which, as already mentioned, is increasingly proving to be an important communication tool in community health education. The following description (Box 17) is an innovative example (Soegijoko 2009) of how such appropriate ICTs, either alone or in combination with other technologies, are actually being applied in settings like the health centres and community clinics where, as we mentioned earlier, relevant community health practice, research and education can be undertaken in a cooperative and collaborative manner.

As can be seen, this account includes the possibilities of using various ICT applications that may not all be traditional and cheap. Although we have in the foregoing discussion in especially Part Two, Chapter 9 (Tables 3 and 4) considered the

**Box 17: Mobile Telemedicine System for Ambulance and Movable Community Health Centre**

"Since 2005, special efforts have been dedicated to the development of "mobile telemedicine system with multi-communication links". Basically, the mobile telemedicine system consists of a base unit (to be installed in a hospital or healthcare unit) and a mobile/movable unit (to be installed in an ambulance or in a movable vehicle). The system has been designed to select an acceptable (existing) communication link at a particular location of the mobile (or movable) unit. The system can measure and transfer different types of medical information (e.g. ECG signals, blood pressure, temperature, etc ) from the mobile (movable) unit to the base unit. Two prototypes have been produced and successfully tested; one set (pair) of prototype will soon be installed in Sukabumi (West Java). Different types of existing telecommunication infrastructure can be automatically selected, thus the term "multi communication links".

*Source: Soegijoko (2009)*

benefits of ICT-supported learning, we have also outlined the many drawbacks in using new ICT tools to enhance learning in the community. As already mentioned, most new technology training methods can be superior to traditional methods because a positive learning environment can be built into the method. But as we have also seen development costs of new technology education and training methods are high. Considerations include funds for development, geographic dispersion of trainees, trainees' difficulty in attending training, and whether new technologies are part of the health unit's business strategy. Reviewing the advantages and disadvantages, facilitation strategies, facilitator and student roles, and delivery methods will provide the student with enough information to make an educated decision about the best path for him or her. Online community health facilitators should follow the same procedure of which method of instruction is preferred.

We know that technology changes rapidly, and newer, more cost-effective and more powerful technologies will continue to emerge for potential use in community health education. At the same time, evidence shows that, once installed in schools, ICTs continue to be used for the life of the functioning life of the technology, whether or not newer, more cost effective and powerful technologies emerge (especially as upgrade paths are seldom part of initial planning).

Much of the publicly available information about the effectiveness of particular ICT tools is generated by the companies that market such products and related services.

Applicability of ICTs in developing countries and in particularly the decentralised professional development/continuing education in settings like health centres and community clinics where professional development is provided at the local level of PHC demands much more thought. While it is clear that it is the application of various ICTs that are the most important determinants of the effectiveness of such tools in education, the choices of tools, as we have seen, are quite varied and each has its own advantages and disadvantages. Policymakers and donor staff are often bombarded by information and studies from vendors on the suitability of their products or services, and there is a need for further, independent research on the appropriateness of specific tools with potential to help meet education-related MDGs, for example.

There is need for further investigation and research into the use of ICT for professional development/ continuing education at particularly the local level of PHC. Such research should look at (Prucano 2005):

- the types of models that exist for the effective utilisation of ICTs to support ongoing professional development for educators.
- the best practices for mainstreaming pilot projects involving interactive radio instruction (IRI) in community health, particularly at the local level, and how such projects are managed and maintained over time.
- where computers should reside in, for instance, health centres and clinics if they are to have the greatest learning impact in community health education.
- whether or not the use of ICTs, as in-clinic or health centre presentation instruments, is a cost-effective use of technology.
- approaches to using handheld devices, including SMS-enabled mobile phones, to support education, especially education connected to the professional development of teachers and community health school administration, and what the emerging best practices are.
- approaches to using existing community and interactive radio networks outside the education sector to benefit community health education.
- the successful models that exist for opening ICT facilities in schools to the wider community.
- whether the use of so-called "open source software" offer compelling benefits in education.
- the models that exist on effective public-private-community partnerships in education for ICT equipment provision and maintenance.

Concerning global initiatives and regional networks to enhance literacy and continuing education in community health, the need for synthesis and publication to further enhance advocacy and capacity building in the field of adult education in particularly the community health systems of developing countries cannot be overemphasised. Perhaps of all the conference conclusions, this is an area that is lacking and requires most attention. Developing countries share not only the problem of inefficient and ineffective health information infrastructure but also the difficulty of using health data for planning. The reporting system should include international, regional and national networks, as well as strengthening sub regional cooperation to promote exchange and sharing of ideas, experiences and resources. Countries need to encourage more discussion on their standards and policies of membership, an accepted definition of CLCs, and their functions among stakeholders. Countries can use social media such as Skype to link CLCs across countries as they are much easier to use for this purpose, and for the wide promotion of mutual learning and information sharing among CLCs. The WHO Regional Offices, such as AFRO for example, can function as a platform to collect documents and materials for knowledge sharing, as a discussion forum in members' countries and to help accelerate programmes to meet the community health literacy goals in the health regions.

**Summary**

This chapter dealt with the issue of developing teaching and learning centres in community health education. First, the chapter outlined various types of teaching and learning centres in both developed and developing countries. It then focused on development of teaching and learning centres that are best suited to the needs of Community Health/PHC education, stressing the importance of TLCs that are located in decentralised systems of PHC. Finally, the chapter described a teaching and learning centre design strategy that agrees with the concepts and principles of community health/PHC and is appropriate to local circumstances.

The following final chapter presents the conclusions of this book.

# 14

## *Conclusions*

The main purpose of this book is to demonstrate how faculty, students and communities can engage and learn from each other in order to re-build community and enhance learning in community health through three strategic community processes of designing learning spaces, using information, communication technology, and designing pedagogy, curricula and co-curricular activities for learning. The book also aims to emphasise the important role ICT- supported cooperative and collaborative learning can play in fostering a community of learning in community health and how community health educators can use these learning approaches to enhance such learning. The book is divided into two parts. Part One contains a set of theories, models, concepts and frameworks for enhancing understanding of the three strategic processes of building a community of learning. Part Two seeks to show how the theories, concepts, etc, can be used to help understand the issues that influence the building of a community of learning. We now present conclusions on the set of theories, models, concepts and frameworks outlined in Part One.

**Concepts**

The chapters in Part One looked at:

- Community health and primary health care
- Traditional and new educational theories and ideologies
- Curriculum and curriculum models
- Learning theories, concepts and principles
- ICTs and learning in the community
- Leadership and management theories
- Building of a community of learning framework

We argued explicitly or implicitly in these chapters that theories of behaviour are crucial for organisation design. The set of theories, models, concepts and frameworks outlined in Part One includes mainly conceptions about behaviour and organisation design. But tradition is as important to organisational design as any underlying theory, as the chapters of the book demonstrate. For example, until recently, no one had questioned the predominance of the medical model (the traditional approach to the diagnosis and treatment of illness as practised by physicians in the Western world since the time of Koch and Pasteur) in health care. Such tradition, as we have seen, has particular implications for building a community of learning in community health. Not only are health disciplines partitioned, institutions are organised in ways that do not encourage community. In health educational institutions tradition encouraged specialists to attend to their individual areas, such as faculty developing pedagogy and curriculum exclusively. We have seen that most community health schools have developed community-oriented experiences for their students to prepare them for their roles in community health. However, these community health experiences located in clinical practice settings far away from the colleges and universities fail to completely involve the community in their design. The chapters have shown that what is needed now and in the 21st century in community health education is the development of educational provisions such as learning spaces that encourage communication aided by ICT rather than distance.

However, what the chapters have demonstrated more than anything else is the particular crucial role concepts play in organisation design. The concepts we have covered if properly understood should help community health educators explain the past, understand the present, predict the future, have more influence over future events, and experience less disturbance from the unexpected. We have seen that changing values in health systems linked to a changing technology will influence present assumptions of what is sensible organisationally, and that what has been held to be forever valid may prove to be only partially true. This can result in confused and discontinuous change, which suggests that one should not manage future organisations on past assumptions.

These are examples of assumptions that seem to be losing their value in community health education:

- Lecture theatre
- Hierarchy is natural

**Assumptions that appear to be gaining importance are:**

- Learning in small groups carrying-out problem-solving cooperatively
- The communications revolution
- Flexibility
- Team-based learning
- Transfer of learning
- Lifelong learning
- Learning communities
- Display technologies
- Interactivity
- Distance learning
- Computer-based testing

- Lecture cast (audio-video)

We have also seen that, just like ideas, technologies, etc, organisations and the assumptions on which they have been created, have life cycles. They grow then decline. What this means for community health education systems and organisations, which the chapters have shown, is that the survival and prosperity of these systems and organisations will depend on their ability to do away with old ways of doing things and adopt new modes. The implications of all these are shown in Part Two which tries to demonstrate how the concepts can be used to better understand the issues that influence the building of a community of learning via the three community strategic processes of designing learning spaces, using information, communication technology, and designing pedagogy, curricular and co-curricular activities for learning, on which we now make these conclusions.

**Learning Space Design**

There is an urgent need in the 21st century in community health education for new learning places that foster information exchange between all stakeholders in the process of preparing professionals for their roles in community health. Designing learning spaces should be a process of discussion and innovation that includes facilities manager, faculty, student development professionals, administrators, architects, students, technologists and other stakeholders. This is required to develop spaces that would enhance interaction between students and staff in the teaching and learning process. It is this plural perspective that the intricate nature of projects carried out by students demands to provide the needed information for arriving at informed decisions that team learning requires. Health educators seldom have the chance to participate in the forming of new physical learning spaces be it renovating an existing space or creating new building designs. But, given the chance, health educators can develop or participate in the development of encouraging locations that foster and improve the unique teaching and learning strategies the foregoing chapters have considered, particularly the cooperative and collaborative learning modes.

The need to train more health professionals for the complex and ever-changing community health systems should particularly drive the design of new learning spaces on health professional training institutions and the community where they are to function. This is why community health educators who are often inexperienced concerning construction project are being required to participate in the development and implementation of these new spaces. Community health educators should engage with other construction team members, including information and educational technologists, architects, building planners and learners to harness their expertise and ensure a common understanding. This collaboration is critical to creating spaces that are convenient for teachers and students to use, as well as enhance the achievement of present and future learning goals. This, as we have seen, is particularly challenging in many developing countries because of the complexity of the community health spaces, such as the clinics and health centres. To accommodate especially the healthcare realities and the new teaching strategies of cooperative and collaborative learning, the pedagogical, curriculum and co-curricular activities of both teachers and students in the community will continually demand increasingly sophisticated facilities that can facilitate community of learning and provide for the kinds of education that are associated with community of leaning, such as interdisciplinary learning.

This means that community health educators should consider in the learning space design process the kinds of pedagogical and curriculum approaches to fostering community of learning, as well as how to design the learning environment to foster community of learning, based on these pedagogical and curriculum approaches. This requires consideration of the changes in healthcare and educational systems that are needed to design learning environments that suit the pedagogical and curriculum approaches and meet the requirements of a community health/ PHC-centric education. These considerations include in particular development costs, the professional orientation of the setting where learning spaces are to be designed, the scope or location of the learning environment to be designed, the management style in the various community health agencies where learning environments are to be designed, the type of organisation that is involved in learning environment design, patient/client accessibility to health services provided by public, private or voluntary health services, and the need for trainees to be aware of local communities, and to be able to work in and within such communities.

**Technology, communication and information exchange**

The preceding chapters have shown that many new technologies, such as the Internet, have features that help to ensure learning and transfer of training. These features include self-pace, the ability to appeal to multiple senses, finding information from experts on an as-needed basis and receive feedback and reinforcement. New technologies also make it possible for community health professionals to participate in education and training from home or work for several hours. Students do not only control the presentation of educational provisions but also the place and time they participate in education and training. Different new technologies are designed to be used in various places and ways to achieve different learning outcomes. For example, technologies such as virtual reality can create a more realistic training environment, which can make the material more meaningful and increase the probability that training will transfer learning to the job. The chapters have shown the superiority of most new technology training methods over traditional methods because a positive learning environment can be built into the method. However, development costs of new technology training methods are high, including expenses for development. Also, there are other considerations, such as whether new technologies are part of the health organisation's business strategy, geographic dispersion of employees, and trainees' difficulty in attending training,

The previous chapters have demonstrated that despite the challenges and problems faced in developing and implementing ICT applications in community health, the outcomes are in general very promising and encouraging. There is, however, the need to further develop and implement activities qualitatively and quantitatively multiplied in order to enhance the implementation of ICTs widely in community health centres and clinics. This requires the involvement of government institutions, private industries (as part of their corporate social responsibility), and the whole community in efforts at implementing sustainable ICT-supported learning in community health. Such stakeholders must give attention to human resource and human resource development for e-Health, continuing supports in terms of policy, funding, and technical support, availability of ICT infrastructure, and capital and operational costs.

Generally, the use of ICT to support collaborative group learning has yet to be a common phenomenon in today's classrooms (e.g. Becta, 2007). This is arguably more so in communty health education. Therefore the community health teacher needs to build the culture of collaborative and cooperative learning, both online and offline over an extended period of time. This requires continuous effort and using strategies such as: praising a group for their collaborative effort, demonstrating how different ideas can be combined to build a better idea, assessing the students based on group effort, and showing students how they have progressed as a group over time. Sustained period of professional development is also necessary for teachers to develop the competencies needed for computer-supported community-based learning

To inculcate collaborative learning is culture shifting work that entails changing students' dispositions in learning. As we highlighted in the chapters of this book, cooperative/collaborative learning offers many opportunities for students to acquire important knowledge and skills. It is therefore important for teachers to develop collaborative learning as a core component of their pedagogical skills.

**Pedagogy, Curriculum and Co-curricular Design**

The principles of PHC and community health remain valid today and attempts directed toward the achievement of the "Health for All" goal need to be intensified. Orientation with these principles is central to success in efforts at building a community of learning for community health. The community-centred rules of the goal demonstrate the significance of educating through community to community health educational institutions. The rules must therefore find expression in the design of the pedagogy, curricular and co-curricular offerings to help make a community health-centric goal a reality. Thus, such design needs further consideration. The rational and instrumental approach to planning the education of healthcare professionals that overemphasises the behavioural objectives approach to educational planning cannot adequately meet the educational needs of community healthcare professionals who must deal with a host of socio-cultural, economic, political and other factors that affect and will continue to affect health care and related social systems in the years ahead.

Curriculum planning models, such as the cultural analysis approach to curriculum planning that can incorporate other useful educational planning models and principles, for example the curriculum process model, as well as progressive teaching strategies and methods as proposed in this book will provide the necessary learning. These models will also provide the tools that teachers, who are often overwhelmed by the requirement to orient curricula to community health/ PHC approach, need to be successful in meeting this demand. The cultural analysis approach includes the idea of a common-core curriculum that does not rest upon assumptions about cultural uniformity and consensus, rather a common-core curriculum provides a means of coping with cultural diversity in a positive way (Lawton 1982). Cultural analysis is a tool by which those involved in the planning of curricula can choose from cultural content that will equip all health professionals to comprehend and, if need be, to change the health systems in which they work in positive ways.

A limited or simplified idea of the link between planning pedagogy, curricular and co-curricular activities in community health and implementation produces a significant limitation that must be addressed. Implementation cannot be considered as part of a linear or sequential policy process in which political dialogue takes place during policy formulation, and implementation is undertaken by administrators or managers. The process is far from simple and non-communicational; it is a complicated and interacting process which involves implementers of education, who may actually influence the execution of education policy and should participate actively in the planning of innovation and change. To bring about the needed changes that will accommodate the realities of health care, policymakers, community health training institutions, and professional associations should coordinate planned interdependent change in management systems, policies and resources including human resources. Leadership at all levels must invite people with different perspectives to the table when designing pedagogy, curricular and co-curricular new approaches and making decisions. This will assist community health educators to recognise the value and importance of community as a medium for learning.

This means that there must be a change to a more open and participatory approach to innovation and change if the new curricular approaches we covered in the foregoing chapters are to be implemented most successfully. This should not mean that the linear and sequential problem-solving approach to implementing change must be rejected completely. Community health educators can use the rational-empirical approach when dealing with especially other health professionals, experts, researchers, etc., as this will be a necessary strategy in the change process. But as the evidence in the chapters of this book strongly demonstrates, the interacting and participatory approach to curriculum policy is most likely to produce the best results in most curriculum policy environments, such as the local levels of PHC. Such an approach must rest on a clear understanding and use of, for instance, effective policy analysis processes and techniques which, as we have seen, can usefully be provided by professional development programmes and teaching and learning centres.

Thus, community health educators and their collaborators should experience professional development opportunities that provide them with the opportunity to benefit from traditional training covering important work-related skills, techniques and knowledge, but most crucially learning and personal development, which extend the range of development way outside conventional work skills and knowledge, and creates far more exciting, liberating, motivational opportunities for people and their employers. Learning communities should be created particularly in health centres and clinics at local levels of PHC in faculty and community development programmes, where they can provide a valuable learning process for those engaged in practice, education and research. In these healthcare settings, community health educators and their partners can engage in open discussion and sharing among faculty and other stakeholders in the educational process, as well as dealing with questions that relate to the nature of students and how they can be helped to learn.

Community health educators should advocate the development of Teaching and Learning Centres that can provide strong instruments for advancing change in community health systems in favour of the pedagogical, curricular, and co-curricular approaches the foregoing chapters have dealt with. Health centres and clinics, particularly those at the periphery of healthcare systems, can serve as teaching and learning centres where partnerships between student learning and faculty are advanced, and where faculty are prepared to facilitate learning in community and prompt them to consider the value of co-curriculum in student learning. In such health centres and clinics, community health education leaders, who articulate and implement a community-centric mission, can serve as valuable change agents for the curricular, pedagogical and co-curricular innovations that advance community and change community health schools into more community health learning-centred institutions.

The foregoing chapters have demonstrated that it is critical and possible to build a community of learning for community health through the three strategic community processes of designing learning spaces, using information, communication technology, and designing pedagogy, curricula and co-curricular activities for learning. This is particularly indicated for community health higher education which, as we have seen, often underestimates the value of community approaches. Inspired by Bickford et al (2010) this book demonstrates that a community can and does make a difference when we learn to channel interests and focus people's efforts towards a community health/PHC education-centric mission.

# Bibliography

Adefunmike, A.L (2013). Personal Interview.
Agency for Healthcare Research and quality. (2013). Community health centres integrate rapid HIV screening in to routine primary care leading to significant increases in testing rates. Agency for Healthcare research and quality 2013-05-08
Ahmed, S .(2011). School organisation and management. Retrieved from http://edchat.blogspot.com/ .
Alderfer, C (1972). Existence, relatedness and growth: human needs in organizational settings: Free Press.
American Association of Medical Colleges .(2009). Effective use of educational technology:
recommendations and guidelines for medical educators. AAMC; 2007. Retrieved from https://services.aamc.org/Publications/index.cfm?fuseaction=Product.displayForm&prd_id=1 84&cfid=1&cftoken=2580FE75-FF18-4713-997A7BAA5355EF49. .
American Institute of Architects Best Practices. (2007). Defining the Architects Basic Services. Retrieved from http://www.aia.org/aiaucmp/groups/secure/document/pdf/aiap026834.pdf
American Telemedicine Association. (2006). Telemedincine, telehealth and health Information Technology. Retrieved from http://www. Americantelemed.org/docs/default-so
Anderson, L. W. & Krathwohl, D. R., et al. (Eds.). (2001). A taxonomy for learning, teaching, and assessing: A revision of Bloom's taxonomy of educational objectives. Boston, MA: Allyn & Bacon
Ashley, C and Ntshona, Z (2003) Transforming roles but not reality?: private sector and community involvement in tourism and forestry development on the Wild Coast, South Africa. IDS. Research Paper 6. Sustainable Livelihoods in Southern Africa. Retrieved from http://qhr.sagepub.com. (Accessed 3/6/2013)

Bandura, A. (1976). Self-efficacy: the exercise of control. N.York: Cott-Freeman
Bandura, A. (1986). Social foundations of thought and action: a social cognitive theory. Englewood Cliffs, N,J: Prentice Hall
Balcom, P.A. (2001). Minimalism and beyond: second language acquisition for the 21st Century. Second Language Research 17,3. Retrieved from http://sir-sage pub.com
Beattie, A. (1987). Making a curriculum work. In: Allen, P and Jolley, M, eds. Curriculum in Nursing Education. London: Croom Helm.
Becta. (2007). Harnessing technology: progress and impact of technology. Retrieved from http://publications.becta.org.uk/display.cfm?resID=33979&page=1835 (Accessed 6/6/2008)
Ben-Eli, M.U. (2005/2006). Sustainability: the five core principles. Retrieved from http://www. Sustainability labs.org/page/sustainability
Betancourt J.R., Green A.R., Carrillo J.E., et al. (2003). Defining cultural competence: a practical framework for addressing racial/ethnic disparities in health and health care," Public Health Reports 118, 4 (Jul-Aug 2003): 293-302.
Betancourt, J.R., Green, A.R., & Carrillo, J.E. (2002). Cultural Competence in Health Care: Emerging Frameworks and Practical Approaches. The Commonwealth Fund Field Report. October 2002
Bhatia, M., & Rifkin, S. (2010). A renewed focus on primary health care: revatilise or reframe?. London: Department of Social Policy, London School of Hygiene and Tropical Medicine

Bickford, D.T., Deborah J. B & David J. W. (2010?). Community: the hidden context for Learning. Dayton, USA: University of Dayton. Retrieved from http://www.educause.edu.
Blair, M, Koury, S., De Witt, T., & Cundall, D. (2009). Teaching and training in community child health: learning from global experience. Retrieved from http://ep.bmjjournals.com/content/94/4/123.extract.
Bloom, B. (1956). Taxonomy of educational objectives. Boston USA: Allyn & Bacon
Bloom, B. S., & Krathwohl, D. R. (1956). Taxonomy of educational objectives: The classification of educational goals by a committee of college and university examiners. Handbook I: Cognitive domain. New York: Longmans, Green
Boaden, N., & Bligh, J. (1999). Community-based medical education. New York: Oxford University Press
Boettcher, J. (1997). Pedagogy and learning strategies. Retrived from : http:www.csus.edu/pedtech/Learning.html.\.
Bourdieu, P. (1986). The forms of Capital. In Richardson, J (ed). Handbook of theory and research for the sociology of education, 241-256.
Brown, A.E. (2001). Biographical Dictionary of Management. Tisemmes Press
Bruffee, K. (1995). Sharing our toys: cooperative learning versus collaborative learning. Change 27.1 (Jan-Feb 1995): 12–18.
Burns, J. M. (1978). Leadership. New York: Harper and Row.

Carrol, J.M .(1998). Minimalism beyond the Numberg Funnel. Cambrige, MA: MIT Press
Center for Disease control and Prevention. (2011). What is health marketing ?. CDC 1600 Chfton Rd, Atlanta GA 30333, USA. Available at http://www. Cdc.gov/health communication /tools tem/
Chynoweth, P. (2006). The Built environment interdisciplinary: A theoretical model for decision-makers in research and teaching. Proceedings of the CIB working Commission, building education and research conference, Kowloon Sangri-la Hotel , Hong Kong, 10-13 April 2006
Coleman, J.S. (1988). Social capital in the creation of Human capital. American Journal of Sociology, Vol 94
Collins, C and Green, A. (1994). Decentralization and primary health care: some negative implications in developing countries. Int J Health Serv. 1994;24(3):459-75.
Conlan , J., Grabowski, S and Smith, K. (2003). Adult Learning. In Orey, M. (ed). Emerging Perspectives on learning , teaching and technology. Available at http://projectsicoe.nga.edu/epltt
CQ University.(2011). Learning and teaching education research centre. Retrieved from http://content.cqu.edu.au/FCWViewer/view.do?page=1077 .
Culatta, R. (2013). Minimalism (J. Carroll). Innovativelearning.com. Retrieved from http://www.instructional design.org/theories/minir.
Cuyamaca College (2012). Professional Development. Retrieved from http//www cuyamaca.edu/professional dev/.

Dahlgren, G and Whitehead, M . (2006). European Strategies for tackling social inequities in health. Liverpool: University of Liverpool, WHO Collaborating Centre for Policy Research and Social Determinants of health
Dahlgren, G and Whitehead, M. (1991) Social Model of Health. Available at http://www.nwci.ie/download/pdf/determinants_health_diagram.pdf
Davis, M.T. (2003). Outcomes –Based Education. Scotland: University of Dundee Centre for Medical Education
Department for the Environment, Food and Rural Affairs. (2009). Sustainable Growth.

***Bibliography***

UK: Defra

Department of Education and early childhood development. (2007). Shared facility partnerships: Aguide to good governance for schools and the community. Victoria: Department of Education and early childhood development. VAILABLE AT HTTP://WWW. EDUWEB.VIC.GOV.AU/EDULIBRARY/PUBLIO/PROPMAN/FAC

Department of Health. (2014). Primary and Community Health. Department of health, State Government of Victoria, Australia. Retrieved from http://www.health.vic.gov.au/pch/

Dialogue by Designers. (2012). Dialogue by design: a handbook of public & stakeholder engagement. Retrieved from http://designer.dialoguebydesign.net/docs/Dialogue_by_Design_Handbook.pdf the online engagement design system..

Donaldson, L. (2006). Chapter 2: The Contingency theory of organizational design: challenges and opportunities. In Burton, R.M;Eriksen, B; Hakonsson, D.D;Snow, C.C (2006), X111,284p ISBN: 978-0-387-34172-9

Dooly, M.(2008). Constructing knowledge together (21-45) Extract from Telecollaborative Language learning: A Guidebook to moderating intercultural collaboration online. M. Dooly (ed) 2008 Bern: Peter Lang

Edwards, J., Stanton, P. & Bishop, W. (1998). Interdisciplinary: the story of a journey. Nursing and health care perspectives, 3, 116-117

Eklund, P and Stavem, K. (1990). Prepaid financing of primary health care in Guinea-Bissau: an assessment of eighteen village health posts. Policy research working paper 488. Washington DC: World Bank.

Eraut, M. (1994). Developing professional knowledge and competence. London: The Falmer Press

European Commission DG. (2005). Developing local learning centre and learning partnerships as part of member states target for reaching the Lisbon goals in the field of education and training: a study of the current situation. Leiden, The Netherlands: European Commission, Education and Culture.

Feinberg, T. (2009). Institutional Theory. Retrieved from http:// sample-of-term papers. blogspot.com/20

Fiedler, F. E. (1967). A Theory of leadership effectiveness. New York: McGraw-Hill.

Flinders University. (2013). Curriculum Development: Major phases and outcomes. Flinders University Centre for University Teaching. Innovative

Fonchingong, C.C and Fonjong, L.N. (2003). The concept of self-reliance in community development initiatives in the Cameroon Grassfields. Nordic Journal of African Studies 12 (2): 196-219

Freire, P .(1974). Pedagogy of the Oppressed. New York: Seabury. Translated from the original Portuguese by Myra Bergman Ramos

Friedman, A. L.., Miles, S. (2006). Stakeholders: theory and practice. Oxford: Oxford University.

Gagne and Medsker, The conditions of learning; Howell, W.C and Cooke, N.J. Training the human information processor: a review of cognitive models. In Training and development in organisations,(ed). I. L Goldstein and Associates (San Francisco:Jossey-Bass,1991):121-82

Ghen, D. (? ). A sum of Summaries: Pedagogy of the Oppressed. Retrieved from http:// sum summaries. Tumblr.com/post/41456013682/pedagogy-of-the oppressed\

Giri, K., Frankel, N., Tulenko, K., Puckett, A., Bailey, R and Ross, H. (2014). Keeping up to date: Continuing professional development for health workers in developing countries. WHO: Global Health Workforce Alliance.

Gofin, J & Gofin, R. (2005). Community-oriented primary care and primary health care. American Journal of Public Health, 95(5):757.

Goldsmiths College. (2011). Project governance-Brief Guidance Notes. Retrieved from http://www gold.ac.uk/ project % 20 Governance % 2

Golladan, F.L. (1980). Comnity healthcare in developing countries. Finance Dev, September: 17(3):35-39

Gonzala, A. (2011). The dynamic Nurse-Patient relationship. Retrieved from http://nursing theories. Weebly.com/ida-jean-orlando.ht.

Gonzalo, A. (2011). Theoretical foundations of nursing: the Roy Adaptation Model. Retrieved from http://nursing theories.weebly.com/sister-callister-roy.nt

Good, J. (2013). The Art of saying less: Minimalism. Retrieved from http://www.technicalwritingireland.com/the-art.

Goodin, R. E. (1995). The theory of Institutional Design. Cambridge: Cambridge University Press.

Goodland, R and Daly, H. (1996). Environmental sustainability: universal and non-negotiable. Ecological Applications, 6: 1002-1017.

Goodson, I. & Medway, P. (1975). The Feeling is Mutual. London: Times Educational Supplement.

Gordon, P.A., Campos, J.J.B., Ito, K. and Lima, G.Z .(1998). The challenges of introducing a new curriculum in a traditional environment. In Programme. International conference on partnerships for community health. The Network of Community-oriented educational institutions for health sciences, Albaquerque, New Mexico, USA.

Government of Alberta. (2014). Teachers as Role Models for Healthy Habits. Alberta: Government of Alberta. Retrieved from http://www. Healthyalberta.com/707.htm.

Graff, G. (2003) Clueless in academe: how schooling obscures the life of the mind. New Haven, Conn.: Yale University Press,

Green, L., Mckenzie, W and James F. (2002). Community Health. Encyclopedia of Public Health. Retrieved from Encyclopedia.com: http://www.encyclopedia.com/doc/1G2-3404000207.html.

Green, L.W., and Ottoson, J.M. (1999). Community and Population Health, 8th ed. New York and Toronto: WCB/McGraw-Hill.

Greeves, F. (1984). Nurse Education and the Curriculum. London & Sydney: Croom Helm.

Gretchen, L., Nicholas, W., Watkins, S., and Williams, E. (2011). Online Learning Comparisons: synchronous and asynchronouss learning. Retrieved from http://asynchronous and synchronous learning comparison. W .

Gross, N. (1971). Implementing Educational Innovations: A sociological Analysis of planned Educational change. N. York: Basic Books Inc.

Hampel, R.L .(2008). Progressive Education. The Global Group Inc. Available at http://www. Fags.org/ childhood/ Pa-Re/ programme

Handy, C .(1993). Understanding Organisations. London: Penguin Books LTD.

Haynes, J. (2012). Advantages and disadvantages of asynchronous and synchronous learning. Retrieved from http://asychronous and synchronous learning.blogsp

Haythornthwaite, C. (2005). Building community Networks. Retrieved from http://net.educase/ir/libary/pdf/EQMO848.PDF .

123 Help Me .Com. (2014). Strengths and Weaknesses of McClelland's Acquired Needs theory and Expectancy theory. Retrieved from http://www 123 HelpMe. Com/view.

asp?id=164966
Hirschfeld, M. (1997). Strengthening nursing and midwifery: a global study. Geneva: WHO.
House, R. J. (1996). Path-Goal theory of Leadership: Lessons, Legacy, and a Reformulated theory. Leadership Quarterly, Vol. No. 3
HR-Survey.Com. (2013). Needs Analysis: how to determine training needs. Retrieved from www.hr-guide.com/data/G510.htm.
Hughes, R., Black, C and Kennedy N.P. (2008). Public health nutrition Intervention Management: Stakeholder analysis and Engagement. Dublin: Jobnet Project, Trinity College. Retrieved from http://medicine.tcd.ie/nutritio-dietetics/assets/pdf/1-Intelligence.

Infed. (2010). Curriculum theory and practice. Retrieved from http://www.infed.org/biblio/b-curric.htm. .
Intel World Ahead Programme. (2010). Information, communisation technology is transforming healthcare education in the Philippines. White Paper: Transforming Medical education through ICT. Retrieved from htytp://www.who.int/pmnch/events/partners-forum/ICT
International Fund for Agricultural Development (2011). A guide for project M&E, Section 3. Rome: IFAD
Investopedia .(2013). Human Capital Definition. Retrieved from http://www.investopedia.com/terms/h/humancapital.asp (Accessed 27/11/2013).
Iowa State University. (2013). Facilities Planning & Management. Retrieved from http//www.fpm.iastate.edu/planning/capital_planning_process/design.asp .

Jancloes, M. (1998) .The poorest of first: WHO activity to help the poor in greatest need. World Health Forum, Vol. 19, No3.
Jeguier, N. (1981). Appropriate technology needs political push. World Health Forum, Vol.2, No.4, p541-550
Johnson, D, W and Johnson, R.T. (1987). Learning together and alone. Cooperative, Competitive and individualistic learning (2nd ed)Englewood Cliffs, N.J: Prentice-Hall
Johnson, R.L., Roter, D., Powe, N.R., & Cooper, L.A. (2004). Patient Race/Ethnicity and Quality of Patient-Physician Communication During Medical Visits. American Journal of Public Health, 94(12), 2084-2090.
Johnson, W. (n.d.) Social Learning Theory Strengths & Weaknesses. Retrieved from ehow.com

Kahssay, H.M. (1998). Health centres-the future of health depends on them. World Health Forum, Vol 12, No 2.
Kaplan, S and Ashley, J. (2003). Synchronous and asynchronous communication tools. Retrieved from http://www.asaecenter.org/Resources/articledetail.cfm?itemnumber=13572.
Kaur, A. (2013). Maslow's Need Hierarchy theory: Applications and criticisms. Global Journal of Management and Business Studies IJSM 2248-9878 Vol 3 No 10,pp1061-1064
Kearsley, G. (1994a). Conditions of learning (R. Gagne). [Online]. Retrieved from http://www.gwu.edu/~tip/gagne.html.
Kearsley, G. (1994b). Constructivist theory (J. Bruner). [Online]. Retrieved from: http://www.gwu.edu/~tip/bruner.html .
Kearsley, G. (1994c). Social learning theory (A. Bandura). [Online]. Retrieved from: http://www.gwu.edu/~tip/bandura.html.
Kearsley, G. (1994d). Minimalism (J. M. Carroll). [Online]. Retrieved from: http://www.

gwu.edu/~tip/carroll.html .
Kindig, D and Stoddart, G. (2003). What is population health. Am J Public Health, March; 93(3):380-383.
Knowles, M.S. (1990). The Adult Learner: A neglected species. Houston: Gulf Publishing.
Kokemuller, N. (2015a). Advantages and disadvantages of transformational Leadership. Retrieved from smallbusiness.chron.com/advantages-disadvantages-transformational-leadership.
Kokemuller, N. (2015b). Goal-setting theory advantages and disadvantages. Retrieved from www.ehow.com/facts-5312495-goal-setting-theory-advantages-disadvantages-h
Kuh, G.D. (2005). Student success in college: creating conditions that matter. San Francisco: Jossey-Bass.

Lamberti, P. (2012). The Rotarian, February 2012.
Laurent, C.L. (2000). A nursing theory for nursing leadership. Journal of Nursing Management, 8, 83-87.
Lawton, D. (1983). Curriculum studies and educational planning. London: Holder and Stoughton.
Leadership Central.Com. (2013). Path-goal theory-Robert House. Retrieved from www leadership-central.com/path-goal-theory.htm #ax223/PNjc9Lvs
Learning Sciences and Technologies Academic Group. (2010). Structuring Activities for Transiting from Cooperative to Collaborative Learning. Singapore: National Institute of Education
Levine, R., M. Rosenmoller and P. Khaleghian. (2001). Financial Sustainability of Childhood Immunisation: Issues and options. Global Alliance for Vaccines and Immunisations. Retrieved from http://www, vaccinealliance.org/financing/identity.htn .
Lewis, S and Edwards, J. (2004). A thousand points of light?: moving forward on primary health care : a synthesis of the key themes and ideas from the national primary health care conference, Winnipeg, Manitoba, May 16-19, 2004. Retrieved from http://books.google.gm/books/about/A_Thousand_Points_of_Light.html?id=QSnRlgEACAAJ&redir_esc=y .
Lin, C.S. (2013). Social learning theory Vs Social cognitive theory? ResearchGate. Retrieved from http://www. Researchgate/post/social learning
Lisa De Mesa, H .(2014). Curriculum Models: An analysis. Retrieved from www.acedemia.edu/4657356/curriculum -models
Lisagor, K. (2013). Social Networks. The Rotarian, April 2013
Locke, E.A and Latham, G.P .(1979). Goal Setting: A motivational technique that works. Organisational Dynamics, 8(2), 68-80.
Loepp, F.L. (1999). Models of Curriculum Integration. Journal of Technology Studies, 25(2): 21-25

Management Study Guide. (2013). Expectancy theory of Motivation. Available at http://www managementstudyguide.com/expectancy-theory-motivation.htm
Management Study Guide. (2013). Goal Setting theory of motivation. Retrieved from www.managementstudyguide.com/goal- setting-motivation.htm
Manning, G., Kent, C., and McMillen, S. (1996). Building community: the human side of work. Cincinnati, Ohio: Thomson Executives Press
Maslow, A. H. (1943). A theory of human motivation. Psychological Review, 50(4), 370-396
Massey Centre for Teaching & Learning. (2013). New Zealand: University of New Zealand. Retrieved from https://www.massey.ac.nz/massey/staffroom/teaching-and-learning/centres_tl/ctl/about-us/national-centre-for-teaching-and-learning/national-centre-for-

teaching-and-learning_home.cfm .
Mayberry, R.M., Nicewater, D.A., Qin, H., et al. (2006). Improving Quality and Reducing Inequities: A Challenge in Achieving Best Care. Baylor University Medical Center Proceedings, 19(2), 103118.
McClelland, D .(1978). Managing Motivation to Expand Human Freedom. American Psychologist, 33:201-210
McKenzie, J., Pinger, R and Kotechi, J.E .(2011). An Introduction to Community Health. Canada: Jones and Bartlett Publishers
Mcleod, S. A . (2008). Information Processing. Retrieved from lttp://www.Simplypsychology.org/information processing.htlm
Meisslerm. (2012). Social cognitive theory limitations, strengths and weaknesses. Available at http://meisslem.wordpress.com/2012/06/strengths-and weaknesses (Accessed 1/7/2014)
Merron, J. (1998). Managing a web-based literature course for undergraduates. . Online Journal of Distance Administration. I(IV) Winter. State University of West Georgia Distance Education. Retrieved from Http://www.westga.edu/~distance/merron14.html
Microsoft Corporation. (2014). How scheduling works in Projects. Retrieved from http://office.microsoft.com/en-ool/project-helpt
Ministry of Health & Social Welfare. (2012). National Health Policy 2012-2020 "Health is Wealth". Banjul: MOH&SW
Ministry of Health. (1981). The Gambia Primary Health Care Strategy. Banjul: MOH
Mitleton-Kelly, E. (1997). Organisations as Co-evolving Complex Adaptive Systems. British Academy of Management Systems
Module 1:The Curriculum in Clinical Education (2005). Retrieved from http://furcs.flinders.edu.au/education/postgrad/clinicaled/ HLED9005/moduleO1/mod1-sec .
Moen, A., Andrusyszyn, MA., Iwasiw, C., Støvring, T., Østbye, T., Davie, L., Buckland-Foster, I. Erfaringer med bruk av Internett konferansesystem som del av studiet i sykepleievitenskap. (Experiences with Internet conferencing in nursing science). (2000). Vard i Norden (Caring Sciences in the Nordic Countries), 20(4), 42-45.
Morgan, D.L. (1993) Qualitative Content Analysis: A guide to paths not taken. Qual Health Res. 1993 Feb;3(1):112-21.
Mullaly, Z. (1988). The application of a social health perspective: a shared social worker doctor. Retrieved from http://www.tandfonline.com/doi/ref/10.1080/03124078808550026 #tabModule.
Mullan, F & Epstein, L. (2002). Community-oriented primary care: new relevance in a changing world. American Journal of Public Health, Vol. 92, No 11

National Center on Minority Health and Health Disparities (NCMHD). (2008). Retrieved from http://ncmhd.nih.gov.( Accessed July 15, 2008).
National Health Policy: Health is Wealth 2012-2020 (2012). Banjul: Ministry of Health and Social Welfare
National Healthcare Disparities Report (NDHR). uhttp://www.ahrq.gov/qual/nhdr03/fullreport/index.h tml. 2003. Agency for Healthcare Research and
Quality (AHRQ).
Ngo-Metzger Q, Telfair J, Sorkin DH et al. (2006). Cultural Competency and Quality Care: Obtaining the Patient's Perspective. The Commonwealth Fund. October 2006
Nienhuser, W. (2008). Resource Dependence theory: How well does it explain behavor of organisations. Retrieved from http://www.Lampp-ejournals.de/lampp-verlay-service.
Noe, R. A. (1999). Employee training and development. St Louis: Irwin/McGraw-Hill.

Oblinger, D. G. (ed) (2006) Learning spaces. Educase; 2006. Retrieved from www.educause.edu/learningspaces

One-laptop per Child.Organisation. (2014). Retrieved from http://www.one.laptop.org.

Organisation for Economic Cooperation and Development. (2000). The contribution of human and social capital to sustained economic growth and well-being. Canada: OECD.

Organisation for Economic Cooperation and Development. (2007). Human Capital: How what you know changes your life. OECD Insights. Retrieved from http://www. Oecd.org/human capital howw

Organisation for Economic Cooperation and Development. (2007). What is Social capital?. OECD Insights: Human capital. Retrieved from http://www. OECD.org/37966934 pdf

Orlando, I.J. (1990). Dynamic Nurse-Patient relationship: Function, process and principles. In George, J(ed) Nursing theories: the base for professional nursing practice. Connecticut: Appleton and Lange.

Peters, K.E., Cristancho, S.M & Garces M. (2009). Closing the gap in a generation-health equity through action on the social determinants of health. Education for Health, 22(2):381.

Pfeffer, J and Salancik, G. (1978). The external control of organisations: A resource Dependence Perspectives. New York: Harper and Row Publishers

Pfeffer, J. (1982). Organizations and Organization Theory. Boston: Pitman Publishing.

Piaget, J .(1964). Six psychological studies. New York: Vintage

Plochg, T & Kalzinga, N.S. (2002). Community-based integrated care: myth or must? International Journal for Quality in Healthcare, 14:91-101.

Public health Action Support Team. (2011). Collaborative and Individual Responsibilities for health, both physical and mental: Principles and practice of health promotion. Health Promotion and healthy public policy. Retrieved from www.healthknowledge.org.uk/public-health-textbook/disease-causation-diagnostic/2h-principles

Putman, R.D. (1993). Making Democracy work. Princeton, N.Y: Princeton University Press.

Quinn, F.M. (1995). The principles and practice of nurse education. London: Chapman & Hill.

Ramos, M.B .(1974). Freire's Pedagogy of the oppressed: Summary. New York: Seabury

Rasheed, A .(2012). Behavioural learning theory. Retrieved from http://dhiras heed.glogspot.com/2012/05/ behavioral learning theory

Raths, J.B. (1971). Teaching without specific objectives. Educational Leadership, April, pp 714-720.

Reynolds J, Skilbeck M. (1976). Culture and the classroom. London: Open Books

Richards, R. W. (2001). Best practices in community –oriented health professions education: international exemplars. Education for Health, Vol 14, No 3, 357-365

Richards, R.W. (2000). What does "community-oriented" means anyway?: some thoughts on Zohair Nooman. Education for Health, Vol 15, No.2, 2002, 109-112.

Rotary International. (2012). Elements of a Sustainable Project. The Rotarian, November 2012

Roy, C and Andrews, H.A. (1999). Roy's Adaptation Model (2n edition). Stanford CT: Appleton and Lange

Ruderman, M (2000). Resource Guide to Concepts and Methods for community-based and collaborative problem-solving, Women's and Children's Health Policy Centre, Department of Population and Family Health Sciences, John Hopkins University School of Public Health. Retrived from http://www.jhsph.edu/research centre-and-institutes

Saaty, T. (2012). Decision-making for leaders: The Analytic Hierarchy Process in a complex World. Retrieved from http://books.google-c 1 books ? id=c8kq 5WPF wIVC&printsec=cop

Sabally, S (2013) Interview on Gambia's Regional Health Teams and professional development, April 20th 2013.

Sandhu, D. (2013). Answers to "What are the disadvantages of social constructivism or constructivist. Researchgate. Retrieved from www. Researchgate.net/post/what are the disadvantages-of-social constructivism.

Sanzberro, O., Alvarezde Fulate, N., Jareno, M.,Etxeberria, O and Monterola, U. (2014). Research and Promotion of Free-Software Technology Platforms for Massive openline Technology. Valencia, Spain:Foundation ASmoz. Retrieved from http://library.iated.org/view/sanzberro 2014 Res

Sarr, F and Mason, C. (2008). One Online International Collaborative Community Health Assignment for two RN/BSN Program: How We Did it". Public Health Without Boarders. American Public Health Association 136 Annual Meeting and Expo OCT. 25-29, 2008, San Diego, California.

International Online Collaborative Community health Project.

Sarr, F. (2013). Community-oriented education for health professionals: cultural analysis approach to curriculum planning. Banjul, The Gambia: BOHNJACK Group Ltd

Schaay, N. & Sanders, D. (2008). International perspectives on PHC over the past 30 years. South Africa, Western Cape: University of the Western Cape, School of Public Health

Schmidt, H.G., Neufeld, V.R., Nooman, Z.M. & Ogunbode, T. (1991). Network of community-oriented educational institutions for health sciences . International Medical Education, Volume 66, No 5.

School of Primary Aboriginal and Rural Healthcare. (2009). University of Western Australia. Retrieved from http://www.Sparhe.uwa.edu.au/ (Scott Peck, M.(1993). Meditations from the road. New York: Simon and Schuster.

Scott, W.R. (1995). Institutions and organisations. CA: Thousand Oaks

Seth, V.D. (1998). Development of academic primary health care sites. Cape Town, South Africa: Western Cape Community Partnership Project UWC.

Shah, A. (2013). Structural Adjustment-Amajor cause of poverty. Global Issues. Retrieved from http://www. Global issues. Org/ article/ 3/structural- adjust.

Shapiro, M., Cartwright, C.M. & MacDonald, SM. (1994). Community development in primary health care: an Australian experience'. Community Development Journal, vol. 29, no. 3, pp. 222-231.

Shaw, F.B. (1937). A modern concept of education. Am J Public Health Nations Health. 1937 June; 27(6): 587–589. PMCID: PMC1563192. Retrieved from http://www.ncbi.nlm.nih.gov/pmc/articles/PMC1563192/.

Sing, C.C., Wei-Ying, L & Hornmun, C. (2011). Advancing collaborative learning with ICT: conception, cases and design. Singapore: Ministry of Education

Skilbeck, M. (1976). Ideologies and values, unit 3 of course E20, curriculum design and development. Milton Keynes: Open University.

Skinner, B.F. (1953). Science and Human Behaviour. Simmon and Schuster. Com

Smith, C., Davies, L and Sadler, R. (2013). Assessment Rubrics. GIHE, Griffith University. Retrieved from http://www.friffith.edu.au/-data/assets/pdf file

Smith, M.K (1996) Learning in the community and community learning, The Encyclopae-

dia of Informal Education. Retrieved from www.infed.org/lifelong learning/b-dcom.htm
Sobral, D.T et al. (1978).The Medical School of the University of Brasilia. In: Katz, F.M & Fulop, T., eds. Personnel for Health Care: Case Studies of Educational Programmes. Geneva: WHO.

Soegijoko, S. (2009). ICT applications in e-health: improving community healthcare services towards achieving the MDG 5: roundtable on governance and applications of ICT for achieving the MDGs. Bangkok: The United Nations Conference Centre, 9 – 10 December 2009

Souza, K.H. (2009). Learning spaces in health education: best practices in design. Retrieved from https://www.aamc.org/download/83256/data/learningspaceswhitepaper.pdf

Srinivasan, S., Fallon, L.R and Dearry, A. (2003). Creatng healthy communities, healthy homes and healthy people: Initiating a research agenda on the built environment and public health. Am J Public Health, September; 93 (9): 1446-1450

Steakley, M.E. (2008). Advantages, disadvantages and applications of constructivism. University of Tennessee at Martin. Retrieved from www slideshare.net/meskeakley/advantage.disadvantage-and –application-of-constructivism

Stenhouse, L. (1975). An introduction of curriculum research and development. London: Heinemann.

Stephenson, K.S., Richmond, S.A., Hinman, M.A. & Christiansen, C.H. (2002). Changing educational paradigms to prepare health professionals for the 21st century. Education for Health, Vol.15, No.1, 37-47.

Stoner, G. (1996). Implementing Learning Technology. Learning Technology Dissemination Initiative. Retrieved from http://www.icbl.hw.ac.uk/Itdi/index.html.

Szasz, G. (1969). Inter-professional education in the health sciences. Millbank Memorial subsidize Quarterly 47, 449-75

Tenn, L., Sovaleni, R., Latu, R., Fotu, A et al. (1994). Getting the community involved in developing a PHC curriculum in Tonga. International Nursing Review, 41, 5.

Terbuc, M. (2014). Free/Open source Software in Education. Maribor, Slovenia: Unive rsity of Maribor, Faculty of Electrical engineering and computer science. Retrieved from http://www.or.feri.uni-mb.si/. ZobrazevanjePUBLIK

The Health Foundation . (2010) Complex Adaptive systems. Retrieved from http://www.health.org.uk/public/cms/75/76/313/2590/complx adaptive systems research scan.pdf?real

The World Bank Group. (2001). Decentralisation and subnational regional economies. Retrieved from www1.worldbank.org/publicsector/decentralization/what.htm

Tight, M. (1996). Key concepts in adult education and training. London: Routledge.

Tonga, W.T. (2004). Free/Open Source Software Education. ISBN: 81-8147-565-8. ELSERVIER. New Delhi, India

Trucano, M . (2005). Knowledge maps: ICT in education. Washington DC:Infodev/World Bank.

Tyler, R.H. (1931). Basic principles of curriculum and instruction. Chicago, III: University of Chicago Press.

UCL Institute of Health equity. (2010). Fair society, healthy lives: Strategic review of health inequalities in England post 2010 (the Marmot Review) Retrieved from: http://www.instituteofhealthequity.org/projects/fair-society-healthy-lives-the-marmot-review

Ukaigwe, P. (2013). Personal Interview.

UNESCO. (2012). Community learning centres: Asia-Pacific Regional Conference Report. UNESCO Bangkok: Asia and Pacific Regional Bureau for Education.

*Bibliography*


United Nations Conference on the Environment and Development. (1992). New York: UNCED

University of British Columbia .(2013). Organisational and Operational Context of the UBC Vancouver Centre for Teaching, Learning and Technology. Vancouver: Centre for Teaching, Learning and TechnologyTLT, UBC.University of Melbourne. (2013). General practice and primary health care academic centre. Australia: University of Melbourne, 200 Berkely Street, Parkville 3010 VIC, Australia

University of the Sciences in Philadelphia. (2014). Student participation and Active learning. Retrieved from http://www.usciences.edu/teaching/tips/spah.shtml

Unverzagt, M., Kalishman, S and Urbina, C. (1998). Involving Community Representative in curriculum design/community empowerment. International Conference on Partnerships for community health. The Network of Community-oriented educational Institutions for health Sciences, Albuquerque, New Mexico.

Vroom, V.H. (1964). Work and Motivation. (1964). New York: John Wiley.

Vygotski, L.S. (1978). Mind in Society: The development of higher psychological processes. Cambridge, MA: Harvard University Press

Web. (2012). MidCity adds design, space planning, and furniture at community health's new location. Retrieved from http://www.prweb.com/releases/2012/3/prweb9240437.htm

Weidner, T.G. & Popp, J.K. (2007). Peer-assisted learning and orthopaedic evaluation psychomotor skills. Journal of Athletic training 42, no 1:113-19

Williams, I.(2012). Project Governance. Retrieved from http://www. apm.org.uk/protected.../project% 20 Governance % 20 slides.pdf.

Wolf , K.N. (1999). Allied health professionals and attitudes toward teamwork. Journal of Allied Health, 28, 15-20.

Woodcraft, S. (2012). Social sustainability and New Communities: Moving from concept to practice in the UK. Procedia Behavoural and Social Sciences 68(2012): 29-42. Retrieved from www. Science direct.com

World Commission on the Environment and Development. (1987). Brundtland Report. New York: WCED

World Federation for Medical Education (1988). The Edinburgh declaration. Medical Education 22,481-2

World Health Organisation . (1987).The Ottawa charter for health promotion., First international conference on health promotion, Ottawa, 21 November 1986. Retrieved from http://www.who.int/healthpromotion/conferences/previous/ottawa/en/.

World Health Organisation. (1986). Regulatory Mechanisms for nurse training and practice. Meeting Primary Health Care Needs. Geneva: WHO

World Health Organisation. (2014). The World Health Report 2008- Primary Health Care (Now More then Ever). Geneva: WHO

World Health Organisation.(2008). Closing the gap- WHO report on social determinants of health. Geneva: WHO Commission on Social Determinants of Health. Retrieved from http://whqlibdoc.who.int/publications/2008/9789241563703_eng.pdf?ua=1

World Health Organisation.(2010). Telemedicine: opportunities and developments in member states. Retrieved from http://www.who.int/goe/publications/goe_telemedicine_2010.pdf .

World Health Organization .(1995). Renewing the health-for-all strategy. Geneva: WHO.

World Health Organization. (1978). Primary health care. Geneva: WHO.

World Health Organization. (1986). A guide to curriculum review for basic nursing education: orientation to primary health care and community health. Geneva: WHO

World Health Organization. (2008). Primary health care, including health systems strengthening: report by the secretariat. EB124/8, December 4, 2008.Geneva: WHO Commission on Social Determinants of Health.

## *Index*

Printed in the United States
By Bookmasters